Life

IS

"Less is More"

Somatics

Unity Yoga

Petite Pilates

Basic Ballet Barre

Rhythm Remedy
Natural Nutrition

©2018 by Morwenna Assaf

Published and printed by

Tales1001

Cedar Productions

ISBN: ISBN-13: 978-1522877523

ISBN-10: 1522877525

ACKNOWLEDGEMENT PAGE

In creating this book, I have no one person to dedicate it to or to acknowledge. I have had a very wonderful and lucrative career due to those who have inspired me over the years. They are my peers, my teachers and mentors who have touched and inspired my life. As I sit at the far end of my career and look back over the years I realize how fortunate and blessed I am to have known the people that have come into my life. Many of the greats have passed on and many are still here and still touching my life. Those that are gone I visualize as dancing and playing music in heaven. I acknowledge those that are still here and those gone as I have been fortunate enough to have had the finest training, made the best of friends and had a very wonderful career. It has been a life I would not have changed for anything in the world.

My greatest friend in the world and the one who has both been an inspiration and supported me the most, is my husband and partner in life and art, Walid Assaf. Thank you, Habibi, for believing in me and for being my inspiration in life. I am lucky to have had you in my life all these years.

The rest of my friends, peers, students and associates I thank you for everything. It has been a magic carpet ride from here in the US through UK to Lebanon and from New England, CA and TN I have enjoyed the view. As our lives change and the dance too, I am just happy for the life I have had and the contacts and memories that live in my heart. I believe the angels guide us to our true calling. I thank you from the bottom of my heart.

Morwenna Assaf   DancerAndDancer©

WHY I WROTE THIS BOOK

This book is a composite of years and years of research. It has taken me the 40 years I have been in this dance form to research and check all the possible avenues that are beneficial and the best way to handle teaching and the different facets of dance. As I have aged and find different facts coming to life in the health and life of my loved ones and myself, I realize that knowing dance is not enough. I need to know why and how to be able to keep moving all my life or I will end up just another dancer who gives up due to the aches and pains of arthritis and peripheral neuropathy from the over using of movements.

This book is not complete by any means. It was written to give you an open honest slant on things sometimes it may seem harsh. Like anything in life there is always more to learn. We hope to open your eyes and you will be propelled to learn even more and be more proficient an artist. Instructing is not something you learn in a week or a month or even a few years. It is a lifetime of learning. Even though I now do not take regular classes I am still learning. Dance is like the flow of life that is forever changing. Be open, be focused and never waiver from what you believe. *Morwenna* *Assaf*

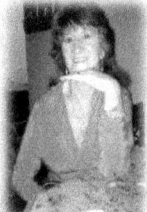

WHAT THIS BOOK IS ABOUT

This book is designed to provide information about the subject matter covered. Which is as listed the basics about Somatic movement, the purpose of Yoga, a small part about Pilates and its purpose plus the addition of basic ballet movements for posture and health. Rhythm Remedy is how to use music and rhythm to your benefit. Plus, Natural Nutrition is about how your food should be based on you and not what others thing. All, of these things, make for a healthy lifestyle to keep you moving forever. It is sold with the understanding that we offer no guarantees as to the outcome.

Humans were made to move. Health is not something that just happens. It takes years, if not a lifetime to accomplish. You must expect to invest time and effort. Life is meant to be lived fully. Be ageless, by being wise in any decisions. After a career in dance, music or anything you live. HOW? By always keeping moving and making wise choices. This book is to help you reach both sides of the coin. It takes dedication and hard work, just like anything else.

Never give up or stop moving

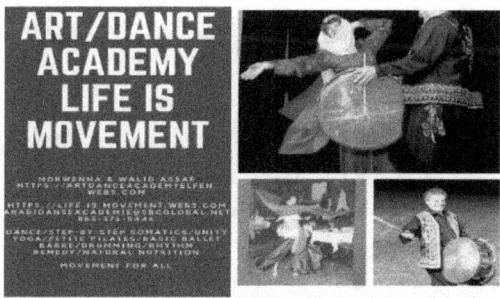

DISCLAIMER PAGE

This book is designed to provide information about the subject matter covered. It is sold with the understanding that we offer no guarantees as to the outcome. Dance, music or health and nutrition is not an easy subject to accomplish. It takes years, if not a lifetime to accomplish. You must expect to invest a lot of time and effort without any guarantee of success.

Every effort has been made to make this book as complete as possible. The purpose of this book is to help give you a lending hand in your health-education so you can, dance, entertain and teach more freely knowing you have some good and well based knowledge under your belt. Neither the author nor the publisher shall have any liability or responsibility to the outcome of studying this book.

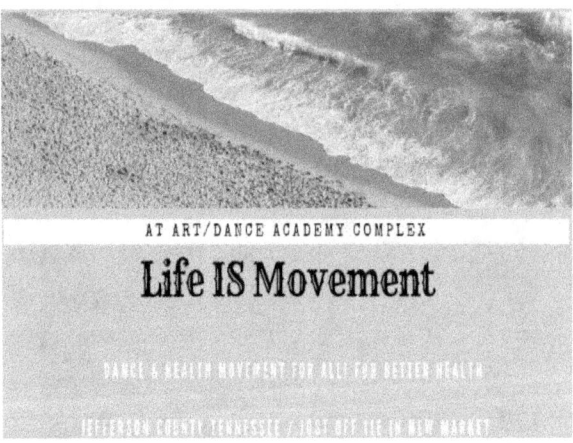

AT ART/DANCE ACADEMY COMPLEX

Life IS Movement

DANCE & HEALTH MOVEMENT FOR ALL! FOR BETTER HEALTH

JEFFERSON COUNTY TENNESSEE / JUST OFF 11E IN NEW MARKET

CONTENTS

RHYTHM REMEDY

NATURAL NUTRITION

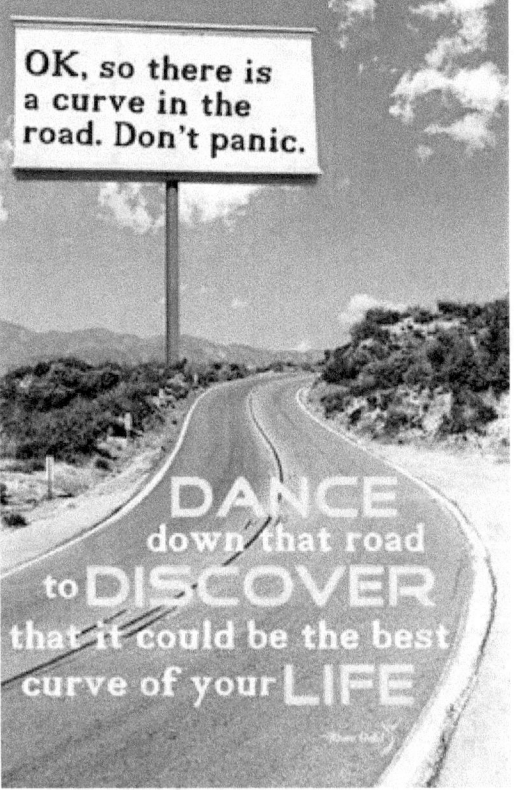

A WORD FROM MORWENNA ASSAF

I have devoted the better part of my life to the wonderful, beautiful dance form called Oriental Dance. It makes no difference what it is called it is a true art form. Even after 40 years giving my soul to it I still love it with the passion I had when I was a younger dancer. I was fortunate to have studied and associated with the finest ever in this business. Now, that my performing days are coming to an end it is time to hit the problems that crop up as time goes by. I have discovered most people come into this dance with no former dance studies and with no concept of this dance as it really is.

My books are a way of sharing what I have learned from the masters of this dance to give you some educated answers to your questions. We have too many people who think dance is instant with no idea of the work involved and the years it takes to be an artist. It is true that to just dance in a nightclub you do not need to be an artist. Being entertaining is often just enough at least for western audiences. Though in reality I do not feel this is true. Even as a club dancer you need background on dance, culture and music. For this dance to have respect in the community you need to have a solid base.

My husband Walid is a premiere percussionist extraordinaire from Lebanon. He has played for renowned dancers worldwide. He has worked with the finest musicians this business has to offer here and in the Middle East. He has devoted his life to this music and dance form. He was born with a *derbecki* in his hand and *debke* in his soul. Yes, we are "Dancer & Drummer"© We now take our knowledge to the next level. That is how can movement and music help the average person in life. Here we help you find the answer. Join us!

BIOGRAPHY OF MORWENNA ASSAF

Morwenna Assaf is the Dance Director for both the Studio and CEDAR Productions. She has been a Middle Eastern (Belly Dancer) dancer, instructor and choreographer for almost 40 years. She studied in New York City with the late Ibrahim Farrah (her mentor and friend), the foremost proponent of the dance in the world. She has continued to study with *Yousry Sharif* America's top instructor of Egyptian dance when he is in CA. Plus she has sponsored and studied the works of the Master Mr. *Mahmoud Reda* of Cairo, Egypt. She has sponsored roughly 6-8 seminars with known names per year. Now cut back due to time constraints.

Even with all the years with "Bobby", Morwenna also studied with other masters of the dance. Although she draws from these other sources, she specializes in teaching the Ibrahim "Bobby" Farrah method, with an emphasis on Middle Eastern folkloric and Danse Orientale (Belly Dancing). Most of the dancers in New England, Kauai, HI and Southern CA namely San Diego County have been trained or influenced by Morwenna and her impact on the dance community has been invaluable. Morwenna also teaches a Gypsy style is called Zambra which is a blend of Rom & Zambra-Mora.

Her forte and that of the dance companies she has run is the Eastern Arabic (The Levant) countries, namely, Lebanon, Egypt, Jordan, Syria and Palestine. Morwenna is a member of NDA, APPHERD, CAPHERD, CID-UNESCO, NDEO and the National Association for Teacher Certification in Middle Eastern Dance – NATCMED. She has taken management courses and seminars with Rhee Gold of MA and belonged to the Dance Studios Mastermind Group with Sam Beckford in Vancouver, BC. She was inducted into the American Middle Eastern Hall of Fame in New York City in 1994 for her contributions, choreography and research in this art form. She was nominated Best Instructor 2001 by Zaghareet.

She has written several books to further the studies of those interested in Middle Eastern Dance Studies. Morwenna has been on the staff of several dance magazines throughout the country. She has written for Gilded Serpent and Take Lessons on Line to share her expertise, on the subject, of Middle Eastern Dance. Has taught dance workshops for CAPHERD for 17 years in both Palm Springs and Riverside, CA. She has also taught for Amani in Lebanon in 2011 with a request' to return again. Every year or so, she does a teaching tour of New England. Plus, Morwenna teaches in Mexico on and Southern CA. Research and writing are at the base of her learning curve at this time.

Morwenna is an internationally known educator. Morwenna has owned and operated her own studio in MA, RI CA and now Eastern Tennessee. She has taught for several esteemed colleges and universities in New England. Plus, Mira Costa College at the San Elijo campus in San Diego North County and maintained her studio in Oceanside CA with her husband, Walid Assaf. Her latest home is located in New Market, Jefferson County, TN.

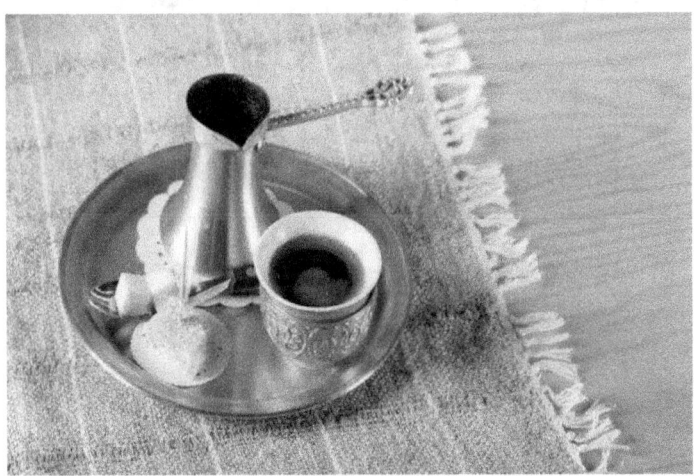

A WORD FROM WALID ASSAF

This book is a culmination of a lifetime dedicated to the dance and music of my country. I have had the pleasure to drum for some of the best dancers in the world. I love this field and hope to transfer those feelings about it to you, the reader. The only way I can express my true feelings, in reality is, by drumming but hope to share what we can through the pages of this book.

Oriental music is in my mind the finest and most complete in the world. It has a complete range from classical to modern pop. Each country has its own variation of modern pop. All are fabulous! Utilize it for your health benefits

Rhythm is fascinating. In Rhythm Remedy we hope to explore all its facets with movement and the mosaic of the rhythms is like stringing together jewels on an interesting piece of jewelry. Open your ears and eyes and feeling to the pulsating rhythm of the percussive drums.

Thank you, *Walid*

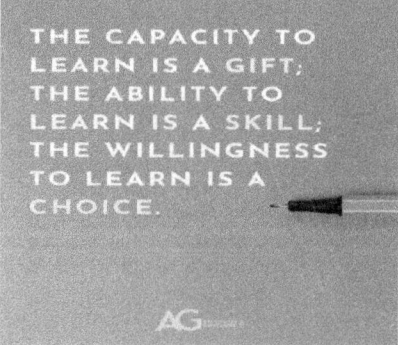

THE CAPACITY TO LEARN IS A GIFT; THE ABILITY TO LEARN IS A SKILL; THE WILLINGNESS TO LEARN IS A CHOICE.

BIOGRAPHY OF WALID ASSAF

Walid Assaf is the Music Director for both Art/Dance Academy and CEDAR Productions. He was known as the leading Arabic drummer of New England and is an artist marked by a very vibrant and energetic style. He shares his skill as an instructor and performer of Arabic percussion. Walid taught percussion through Scheherazade Studios in New England for nearly 20 years then in Southern CA for 18 years He is also a remarkable Debke dancer who brings his talent and knowledge directly from Lebanon. He has performed with the STARS of the dance world on both coasts and in between and in the Middle East. He has performed throughout the world with master musicians and singers from the Middle East.

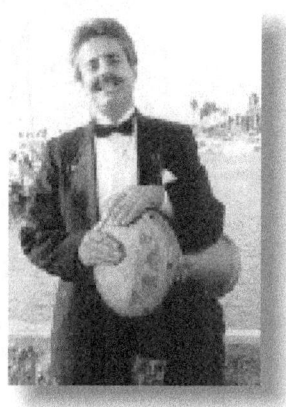

Walid teaches all styles of Arabic percussion including derbecki, tar, table and tambourine. Not only does Walid play several percussion instruments very masterfully, but he is a very qualified DJ dancer, coach and singer. Walid is the manager and directs CEDAR Productions from the publishing. All books CDs and DVDs etc. are written by Tales 1001 but the production of such is done through CEDAR Productions.

His motto is *"Grow like a Cedar of Lebanon"*. This book on understanding the complexity of teaching and performing is a necessary book for all students of Middle Eastern Dance Studies. One cannot separate the culture form the dance or the music. Or the music and rhythm from the soul. This is the best therapy in the world. Along with movement really hear the music.

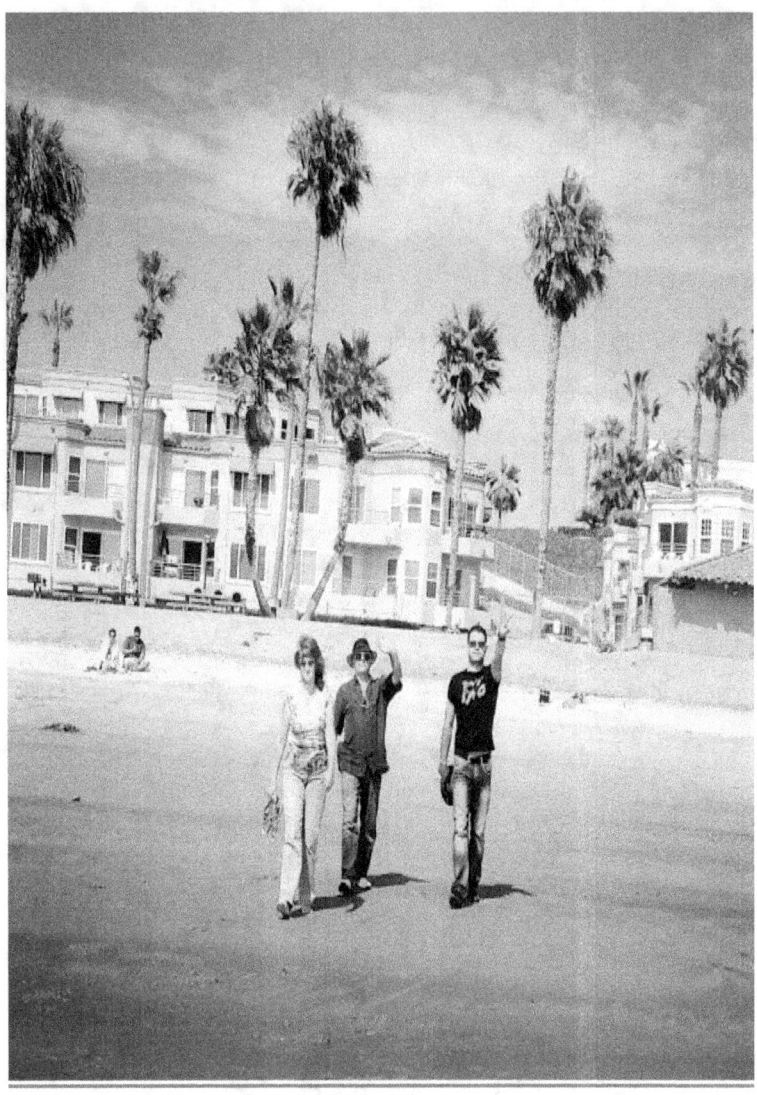

On the beach

Oceanside, CA

Life IS Movement

PART 1:   SOMATICS

For All Stages Of Life

Chapter 1

Middle Eastern dancers and anyone who is physically active in a dance form, gets to the point when their backs, legs and in fact, their entire bodies ache from the years of abuse and exertion. The more prepared you are as a dancer with good technique the longer you will last without pain. But, never the less eventually we all develop pain and aches as we get older. Dancers just last longer than most.

This book is designed for anyone who wants to stay limber and feel well no matter the age or physical capacity. I have danced all my life and am thankful for the great teachers who took the time to share their knowledge and experience that was technique based. I have lasted longer than most but also realize my peers (those who studied with me) are also in excellent shape. We can still run rings around the younger set. We have more energy, do not get as sick as others and prefer to be moving than sitting around.

I notice that as I have gotten older my situation in the dance and how I attack my classes is different than it was say 30 or 40 years ago. I still teach and can still perform. The energy is different, and I might not so aggressive and yes, it has given me longevity. Being a dancer also means I hate exercise. I hate things by rote. Yet these following exercises are relaxing and start my day. I prefer it to yoga which I have found can be boring and, also hard on the body.

It does not take the place of dancing, yoga, body building or other forms of exercise. On days I do not dance I like to walk. But for me even walking becomes boring. So, now I do it with my husband, so we are both benefiting. Our health is most important to us. Yes, we have both retired but we live a very fruitful and interesting life.

We have moved from the San Diego area and now live in Eastern TN. Life is different as we now do not have ocean breezes, forest fires or earthquakes to worry about. But today is the first day of spring and the ground is covered by our first real snow of the winter season. Today is my Habibi's birthday. So, we are housebound. A good day to move forward with this project. We live in a valley at the foot of the Smoky Mountains, so the snow will not last long.

A little on the background of Somatic movement. I come to this as a dance teacher who believes in preserving the body and being able to move comfortably is the best we can do. After reading and studying just about every book there is on the market about dance, health and movement. Because I have a back ailment that has been with me since I was seven years old, I have always

Page16

been very careful of what I do. Thanks to the late Ibrahim (Bobby) Farrah I learned to dance properly and to not harm myself. It has been my crusade, as long as I have been teaching to allow dancers to dance forever and not have physical problems. I know that there is a corner of this dance that says technique is not important to this dance. I say an emphatic no! Dancing technically correct will save your body from harm and also preserves the quality of the dance. No, it is not everything, but technique will also help you acquire the needed results for longevity. So now let us discover how Somatic Movement can help you keep the lasting love for the dance in your life.

Somatic exercise is a study of movement. First let us start with the aging process. As we get older we usually become stiff. Why does this happen? How can we overcome this? Most people believe that aging means degeneration. We may now live longer but are we living better?

The fact is during our lives our bodies respond to daily and yes, dancing stresses. These responses, repeatedly triggered, create habitual muscular contraction. Over use causes them to not voluntarily relax. Eventually this lack of response causes us so that we no longer move about freely. The result is stiffness, soreness and restricted range of movement.

Traumatic accidents or surgery can cause the same reactions. So, this book is not just for the aging dancer but the young also. A program of early training at any age in personal awareness and motor control could help reverse the cause of a whole lot of major health issues. It can change how we live. A great deal can be said of mind over matter. We need and should be responsible for our own actions to help ourselves. This requires education not treatment. It will provide us with a way of living under stressful demands, such as in dance, in a healthy and satisfying way. As we grow older, and we all do, our bodies and our lives should continue to improve as long as we want to.

According to Thomas Hanna the guru of Somatic movement. The human body can be viewed two ways. Looking at it from the outside is what your physician sees. Or what you see when you look at another person. It is just a body, a human shape. But when you look at yourself, it is form the inside with feelings, movement and intentions. A totally different experience. This means being aware. Soma is from the Greek for living body. The human body is then both subjective and objective. To yourself you are soma. To others you are a body. No one can experience or be you. Even when looking in the mirror you are seeing yourself as a body. Only as yourself can you have the privilege of seeing yourself as me.

All human beings need to be self-aware, self-sensing and self-moving. In other words, self-responsible. You can change yourself. In fact, only you can do this. This helps us overcome health problems that are attributed to aging. This allows us to see the whole human being: the self-aware, self-responsible side as well as the observable

Page 18

body side. The complete picture of the human being.

The problems are usually functional not structural. Only you can correct. Not a doctor and not pills. This is caused by loss of control from the inside of the body not deterioration of bodily parts. This is called sensory-amnesia. This is really, non-medical problems. This is caused by the quality of life. It is not the number of years, it is caused by what has happened in those years. Age is neutral as far as health is concerned. Age has never harmed anyone. It is what happens during those years that harms and kills people. This is because everything that happens to us causes a reaction in our nervous systems. Our brain responds and adapts. If we live a restricted, narrow life, our brains react. If we enjoy a a life of confidence and hope, our brains react to that. Our brain does whatever is necessary in order to survive and keep going.

This amnesia affects the entire system and has its roots in the center of the body. Any imbalance in the system creates an imbalance in the entire body. When muscles in one area become restricted or clumsy causes an automatic compensation in interconnected body parts. It has its roots in the center of the body. Namely in the waist, lower back and abdomen. Here are the powerful muscles connect the vertebrae and rib cage to the pelvis. This area is the center of gravity and is the area where signs of "old age" first show up. The muscles in the center of the body are involved, no

Page19

matter what the problem are in the peripheral parts of the body.

"Age" is not the cause of anything "Age" is a neutral term, just like "life". To live is to age.

From our viewpoint this is only part one of a two-part investigation. These problems can be controlled, by relearning. Particularly the muscles of the body's center of gravity need to be addressed.

Slowing down as we age is a death warrant. It is the worst thing we can do. It causes atrophy. Function maintains structure. In other words, use it or lose It! This is the best advice. It is correct, anatomically, physiologically and neurologically. If bones are not used, they become soft. If our muscles are not used regularly they become weaker and less responsive. If our brain cells are not involved in voluntary actions, they deteriorate. This all takes place gradually and insidiously. Not because of aging but because of what we do, or do not do as we age. Bodies break down from deliberate in-action that is built into the way of life. Our brain adjusts to the lack of activity. If certain actions are not part of our behavior, our brain crosses them off. Awareness of how the action was performed fades away. If we reduce our sphere of activity we reduce our chances for health and longevity.

The human body remains adaptive, as long as it is given suitable challenges in which to respond. Regular adaptive physical exercises slow down bone loss and promotes bone growth. Connective tissues shorten if not regularly stretched. Maintaining a broad range physical activity prevents joint stiffness and limited movement. Both the function and the structure of the body declines unless physical activity is constantly maintained. During our middle years, we see the result of the start of impaired motor movement. This includes slower movement, decreased strength and the loss of fine motor coordination. The problem is an inability of the brain to send nerve impulses. This can be corrected by behavioral retraining. This preserves physical fitness. Maintenance of physical fitness through a life-style of daily exercise is an inexpensive and safe method to prevent motor and mental deterioration.

Let us discuss for a minute the front area of the body and how it gets affected. We get a reflex to stressful events. Just living can be stressful. We become overloaded as years go by. So many anxieties in life. This starts at the top and works down. First, we get crows' feet, then a few facial wrinkles, then stooped shoulders etc. down to the knees. It is a with drawl affect. It is burn out. We give in. We have had enough. This then becomes a habitual movement. This involuntary control takes over. We do not function like we used to. It is learned at an unconscious level. This is just on the surface. There are multiple problems going on underneath. We need to keep control.

Somatic exercises are devised to counteract the effects are therapies. They enable us to remember what it feels like to not be anxious, and to breathe and move once again like healthy humans are meant to breathe and move.

Now let us look for a moment the back side of the body and what happens there. Not being conscious of what we are doing is actually negligent, or even irresponsible. 80 percent of adults suffer with back pain. We unconsciously cause our own pain. As we mature and face life and the responsibilities it triggers, the more the back can ache (for example). Within industrial societies of this century adult people habitually contract the muscles of the back. So, we begin to age early in life. Eventually we cease to notice the aches and pains. Just take an aspirin seems to be the answer. We feel fatigue, pain and soreness – in the back of our heads, necks, shoulders, upper back, lower back and butts.

The quality of what happens during our life is way more crucial to our health and happiness than the amount of years we have lived. Reflexes are essential to our survival as humans and as individuals. They are as necessary to us as the air we breathe and the food we eat. The typical problems occur, due, to the effect of muscle withdrawal and the action response. These responses oppose each other, pulling and pushing in opposite directions for mobility and protection. This involves the entire body from head to toe. It also engages the entire nervous system of either withdrawal or positive action. A specific feeling and set sensations accompany this movement. Almost every muscle has an opposite muscle that counterbalances it. This happens in all muscles throughout the entire body. When we contract our bicep to flex our arm the tri-cep automatically relaxes. The front half of the body's muscle contracts while the back half relaxes and lengthens. The idea is like a see-saw balance.

This will not happen as we age if we do not pay attention. Each reflex pattern gradually becomes habitual. At first, just to a small degree but if frequency and intensity increase, the contractions become well established. When one is partially contracted the other cannot contract fully. Muscular mobility by the gradual build-up of opposing contractions. In other words, we are giving in to what is easier. We, have to watch what we are doing because this is the easiest way from major problems to occur.

I do not look like I used to, but I can still do it. This program that I will share with you is where a lot of it **Stiff and Limited Movements**: - Reflexes close in on one another. The skeleton closes in upon itself. The muscles around the body's center of gravity are the central agents of both reflexes. They simultaneously pull the pelvis and hips up towards the trunk, yet, pull the trunk and shoulder girdle down towards the pelvis. All movements become limited. The free rotational movement between the pelvis and the trunk is restricted. This automatically restricts walking. The pelvis does not swing, and eventually the arms lose their counter swing to pelvic rotation. The trunk has become rigid, like a single block. The arms above the trunk and the legs below the pelvis are similarly restricted. Even the head becomes restricted and then it becomes hard to look behind you or twist the head. The arms stop reaching and rotating. Dancing is too much as it is hard to balance and fear of falling develops. This causes people to become more cautious and stiff in their movements. Middle Eastern dancers and anyone who is physically active in a dance form, gets to the point when their backs, legs and in fact, their entire bodies ache from the years of abuse and exertion. The more prepared you are as a dancer with good technique the longer you will last without pain. But, never the less eventually we all develop pain and aches as we get older. Dancers just last longer than most.

This book is designed for anyone who wants to stay limber and feel well no matter the age or physical capacity. I have danced all my life and am thankful for the great teachers who took the time to share their knowledge and experience that was technique based. I have lasted longer than most but also realize my peers (those who studied with me) are also in excellent shape. We can still run rings around the younger set. We have more energy, do not get as sick as others and prefer to be moving than sitting around.

I notice that as I have gotten older my situation in the dance and how I attack my classes is different than it was say 30 or 40 years ago. I still teach and can still perform. The energy now is different and yes, it has given me longevity. Being a dancer also means I hate exercise. I hate things by rote. Yet these following exercises are relaxing and start my

Page 24

day. I prefer it to yoga which I have found can be boring and, also hard on the body.

It does not take the place of dancing, yoga, body building or other forms of exercise. On days I do not dance I like to walk. But for me even walking becomes boring. So, now I do it with my husband, so we are both benefiting. Our health is most important to us. Yes, we have both retired but we live a very fruitful and interesting life.

We have moved from the San Diego area and now live in Eastern TN. Life is different as we now do not have ocean breezes, forest fires or earthquakes to worry about. But today is the first day of spring and the ground is covered by our first real snow of the winter season. Today is my Habibi's birthday. So, we are housebound. A good day to move forward with this project. We live in a valley at the foot of the Smoky Mountains, so the snow will not last long.

A little on the background of Somatic movement. I come to this as a dance teacher who believes in preserving the body and being able to move comfortably is the best we can do. After reading and studying just about every book there is on the market about dance, health and movement. Because I have a back ailment that has been with me since I was seven years old, I have always been very careful of what I do. Thanks to the late Ibrahim (Bobby) Farrah I learned to dance properly and to not harm myself. It has been my crusade as long, as I have been teaching to allow dancers to dance forever and not have physical problems. I know that there is a corner of this dance that says technique is not important to this dance. I say an emphatic no! Dancing technically correct will save your body from harm, and also preserves the quality of the dance. No, it is not everything, but technique will also help you acquire the needed results for longevity. So now let us discover how Step by Step Somatic Movement can help you keep the lasting love for the dance in your life.

Somatic exercise is a study of movement. First let us start with the aging process. As we get older we usually become stiff. Why does this happen? How can we overcome this? Most people believe that aging means degeneration. We may now live longer but are we living better?

The fact is during our lives our bodies respond to daily and yes, dancing stresses. These responses, repeatedly triggered, create habitual muscular contraction. Over use causes them to not voluntarily relax. Eventually this lack of response causes us so that we no longer move about freely. The result is stiffness, soreness and restricted range of movement.

Traumatic accidents or surgery can cause the same reactions. So, this book is not just for the aging dancer but the young also. A program of early training at any age in personal awareness and motor control could help reverse the cause of a whole lot of major health issues. It can change how we live. A great deal can be said of mind over matter. We need and should be responsible for our own actions to help ourselves. This requires education not treatment. It will provide us with a way of living under stressful demands, such as in dance, in a healthy and satisfying way. As we grow older, and we all do, our bodies and our lives should continue to improve as long as we want to.

The human body remains adaptive, as long as it is given suitable challenges in which to respond. Regular adaptive physical exercises slow down bone loss and promotes bone growth. Connective tissues shorten if not regularly stretched. Maintaining a broad range physical activity prevents joint stiffness and limited movement. Both the function and the structure of the body declines unless physical activity is constantly maintained. During our middle years, we see the result of the start of impaired motor movement. This includes slower movement, decreased stressful events. Just living can be stressful. We become overloaded as years go by. So many anxieties in life. This starts at the top and works down. First, we get crow's feet, then a few facial wrinkles, then stooped shoulders etc. down to the knees. It is a with drawl affect. It is burn out. We give in. We have had enough. This then becomes a habitual movement. This involuntary control takes over. We do not function like we used to. It is learned at an unconscious level. This is just on the surface. There are multiple problems going on underneath. We need to keep control.

Somatic exercises are devised to counteract the effects are therapies. They enable us to remember what it feels like to not be anxious, and to breathe and move once again like healthy humans are meant to breathe and move.

Now let us look for a moment at the back side of the body and what happens there. Not being conscious of what we are doing is actually, negligent or even irresponsible. 80percent of adults suffer with back pain. We unconsciously cause our own pain. As we mature and face life and the responsibilities it triggers, the more the back can ache (for example). Within industrial societies of this century adult people habitually contract the muscles of the back. So, we begin to age early in life. Eventually we cease to notice the aches and pains. Just take an aspirin seems to be the answer. We feel fatigue, pain and soreness – in the back of our heads, necks, shoulders, upper back, lower back and butts.

The quality of what happens during our life is way more crucial to our health and happiness than the amount of years we have lived. Reflexes are essential to our survival as humans and as individuals. They are as necessary to us as the air we breathe and the food we eat. The typical problems occur due, to the effect of muscle withdrawal and the action response. These responses oppose each other, pulling and pushing in opposite directions for mobility and protection. This involves the entire body from head to toe. It also engages the entire nervous system of either withdrawal or positive action. A specific feeling and set sensations accompany this movement. Almost every muscle has an opposite muscle that counterbalances it. This happens in all muscles throughout the entire body. When we contract our bicep to flex our arm the tri-cep automatically relaxes. The front half of the body's muscle contracts while the back half relaxes and lengthens. The idea is like a see-saw balance.

This will not happen as we age if we do not pay attention. Each reflex pattern gradually becomes habitual. At first, just to a small degree but if frequency and intensity increase, the contractions become well established. When one is partially contracted the other cannot contract fully. Muscular mobility by the gradual build-up of opposing contractions. In other words, we are giving in to what is easier. We have to watch what we are doing because this is the easiest way from major problems to occur.

Stiff and Limited Movements: - Reflexes close in on one another. The skeleton closes in upon itself. The muscles around the body's center of gravity are the central agents of both reflexes. They simultaneously pull the pelvis and hips up towards the trunk, yet, pull the trunk and shoulder girdle down towards the pelvis. All movements become limited. The free rotational movement between the pelvis and the trunk is restricted. This automatically restricts walking. The pelvis does not swing, and eventually the arms lose their counter swing to pelvic rotation. The trunk has become rigid, like a single block. The arms above the trunk and the legs below the pelvis are similarly restricted. Even the head becomes restricted and then it becomes hard to look behind you or twist the head. The arms stop reaching and rotating. Dancing is too much as it is hard to balance and fear of falling

Page29

develops. This causes people to become more cautious and stiff in their movements.

1. **Chronic Pain**: - Stiff contraction of the body's muscles causes a chronic ache in these muscles. They become sore, sometimes just plain painful. Discomfort in the lower back and pelvic region. These can be from a dull ache to real pain depending on the degree of stressful activity. Restrictions of the shoulder or the hip joints will cause varying degrees of discomfort depending on the kind of habitual activities one engages in. Typists, for example, typically suffer from sore shoulders and necks. Postal workers, sore butts and hips. Pain in the elbows, hands, knees or feet is often mistakes for arthritis, pinched nerves etc.

2. **Chronic Fatigue**: - Being in pain results in an enormous expenditure of energy. Being tired is not the problem. The problem is, one is constantly living with aches and pains. This continues even when lying down and even during sleep. Not only do the muscles ache but you are tired also. This is referred to as fatigue or muscle weakness. No, not weak muscles but strong from constant contraction.

3. **Chronic Shallow Breathing**: - Combining the contractions of the withdrawal and action responses, the rib cage is pulled down both front and back and immobilizes the chest. This provokes shallow, rapid breathing and hyperventilating plus the effects cardiovascular

Page 30

functions. The result is depression, listlessness and loss of mental activity.

4. **A Negative Image**: - These individuals usually develop a negative self-image. They cannot reverse the loss of their youthful functions. Especially if they are constantly told, it is age.

   Causes:
   1. When, you can no longer do what you once could do.
   2. Always in pain.
   3. Tired and without energy.
   4. Oxygen is restricted.

5. **Chronic High Blood Pressure: -** Because of the above listed complaints Hardening of the arteries jumps in. This restricts blood flow.
   1. This causes smooth muscle walls to contract.
   2. The vascular walls are not kept supple or adaptable to blood pressure changes.

There are two ways which muscles work 1. Statically & 2. Dynamically. Static contraction of muscles occurs in isometric exercises. One muscle working against another. Not a good idea. Raises blood pressure.

We are not helpless though. We can avoid the effects of stress. Be aware of stress. We cannot avoid stress, we can control our response to them. Humans are not just a higher being of animal. A human is self- aware and capable of learning greater self-awareness and greater self-control. Recognize, this power. We can save ourselves

Page 31

from the inescapable forces of stress. We can confirm to ourselves the power of human self-responsibility and autonomy – a power that has a much deeper significance.

Solutions are unsuccessful! 99% of the cases of lower back pain are located in the muscles connecting the spine to the back of the pelvis. The pain can be in the lower back or the pelvis, sometimes both. The muscles are painful for one single reason, excessive contraction.

The typical curve in the middle of the body, is not due to a weak back or weak belly. Nor is it due to a structural breakdown. It is due to a chronic involuntary contraction of the back muscles. The problem is in the brain where the reflex is habituated. When this reflex is mastered, the curved back, the protruding belly etc. all disappear, and the pain does too. Sensory – motor amnesia causes us to forget what it feels like to be relaxed, therefor, the distorted back. After years the effects one's sense of straight is distorted. It takes a few weeks to become accustomed to having a tall undistorted back. It is crucial to keep this in mind as you begin to relax and gain a posture that is so much better with, no pain and a more youthful look.

When we are stung by a bee we flinch – this is a trauma reflex. If your body is injured, the cringing is meant to help by providing a protective pattern around the point of injury- this is also a trauma reflex. These kind of trauma reflexes can occur anywhere in the body. This can often affect the smoothness of walking and the sense of balance.

When there is scoliosis, it means a trauma has occurred. Scoliosis can be a simple C curve of the spine or an S curve. An injury has occurred causing the muscles of the pelvis and lumbar spine to contract tighter on one side. Whether the curve is C or S shaped, the cause is usually the same, trauma to the body, causing muscle reflex contraction. The trauma reflex pattern can be caused by severe damage to the body. It can be triggered by surgery. A spastic cringing reaction will occur in the muscles surrounding the site of surgery. Examples of this are endless. It is a reflex to avoid pain.

I have been told since a child that I had one leg shorter than the other and hence scoliosis. The truth is that the muscles of the center of the body were chronically contracted, pulling up the hip on the other side. Inequality of the two sides is very common.

Sciatica is caused by disk pressure on the sciatic nerve. They are sensory nerves, extending through the pelvis, down the thigh and into the feet to the toes. If the pain is moderate, it is felt in the pelvis and hip. If the pressure is severe, it can go all the way to the hip. Nerve pain feels different to nerve pain. It can occur at any age. Sciatica can either be avoided or remedied.

The near miraculous capacity of the human consciousness and the central nervous system can

Page33

learn to adapt. We are capable of far more than we believe we are. As we learn more about the ways the brain functions, control, repair, maintenance and protection are available to us. We also gain more respect for the capacity we have. We are far less dependent and helpless than we believe. We can be far more responsible and self-governing than we know.

Persons with flexible personalities are more likely to continue to perform at high ability levels as they age. In addition to having a flexible style personality, two other conditions are at work. First, a favorable, less stressful personal life and second freedom from arthritis and cardiovascular disease. I find that use- it or lose-it is a principle that applies not only to the muscular maintenance of flexibility but also the maintenance of a flexible life style is related to a high level of intellectual performance as well.

"Expectation" is one of the most important words in the English language. We live in constant change. Living and aging are two identical events. Lives constantly change from the present to the future. The course of our lives follows our expectations in the same way a car drives down the street. The expression "self-fulfilling prophecy" means we get what we wish for. Remember, be careful what you wish for. Why? Because, what we expect to happen, usually turns out to be what happens. Expectation directly contributes to making it happen. Human consciousness is an integral part of the human body's self-regulation.

The attributes beliefs we have about our bodies vitally affect the ongoing state of our bodies and health. If we expect our bodies to be healthy and resilient, they will tend to remain so. If you don't then the opposite can become possible and breakdown will occur. The prophecy is self-fulfilling. We expect it to happen and it will. As we feel certain discomfort, how we interpret them becomes crucial. The feeling of giving-in to an ailment immobilizes our self-healing capabilities. We habitually cringe in response to bodily discomfort, expecting the worst. We are reinforcing the discomfort as a permanent condition. This then becomes resistant to improvement. It can also be an active cause of disease. Respond intelligently with positive countermeasures and awareness. We can directly prevent the disease process, injury, or dysfunction becoming a permanent condition. With the correct attitude we can improve our bodies and the effects of aging will, by and large, not occur.

Age simply means a period of existence. Its root means to grow-up. So, aging can mean either growth of degeneration. Our lives are neither programmed or predictable. Human life is not fixed, it is open. A human life can unfold in the direction of growth and increasing strength, or it can go the other way and unfold in the direction of decay and steady degeneration. Which would you prefer? That is to grow or to decay? If, you want to continue to advance and strengthen then that is more than likely what you will get. Wondering what to expect? Fifty years may be too late. Time is the currency of your life. How you expect to spend it is up to you. What you invest in life is what you will get out of it. Signs of pain etc. are typical adjustments that all bodies go through in regulating and readapting to the future. Aging is an ongoing growth having power to overcome ailments, surmount malaise and defeats of the worst of things. Do not accept failure, do not give up. Drink from the well of life's richest nourishment and wisdom. Life is ever redemptive and rejuvenating.

Have pride in aging. Worshipping youth is the backside of hating advancing age. This attitude is ever popular, unfortunately. Everyone one wants the look and feel of youth. This makes the aging process so much harder. This is ignorant of the nature of life. Youth is not a state to be preserved but a state to transcend. Youth has strength but does not have skill. Youth has speed but not efficiency. Youth is quick but not deliberate and deliberation is the only way to correct bad decisions. Youth has energy and intelligence but not the judgment to make use of it. Youth has beauty but not the beauty of real achievement. Youth has the glow of promise but not the radiance of accomplishment. Youth is a time of planting seeds but not the time of harvest. Youth is a state of ignorance and innocence but not a state of knowledge and wisdom. Youth waits for fullness. Youth is all about explosive yearning. By growing older we transcend ourselves. We are designed to grow by aging. We must remind and re-educate ourselves to the full possibilities open to us. We have blindly ignored the discoveries that can make life and aging a process of growth, achievement, satisfaction and pleasure.

Fear of aging is a product of ignorance. It is time to reverse our traditional superstitions about aging. We need to be more self-conscious and self-regulating. Be educated in how to be controlling the process of our own lives. It is possible to have the body and life that are lasting sources of productivity in satisfaction and pride. Have the pride of age restored back into your life. Be happy, with the promises to be fulfilled. Learn from our youth as a beckoning promise of happiness and fulfillment. Have an attitude of positive expectation. Expect the best out of your life at every birthday. Avoid the ago-old plague of sensory amnesia. Move yourself forward into the future. Make your future the way you want it to be. Life is a continuous process of growth and optimism.

Silence and concentration assist our brain cells to operate in complete balance. It assists the heart to open and will be at one to operate the brain. To create change in the world we, have to change inwardly first.

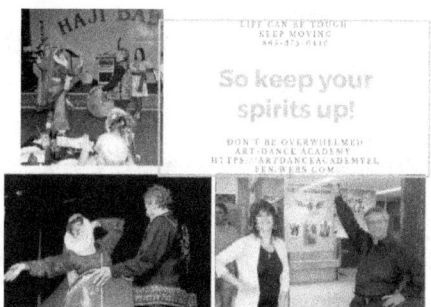

THE HUMAN MUSCULAR SYSTEM

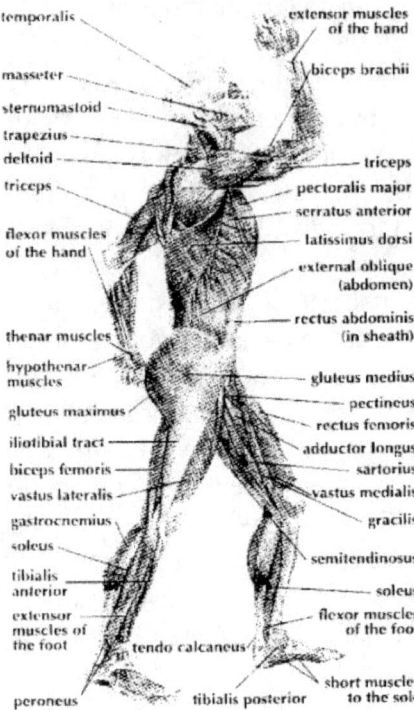

Chapter 2   SOMATICS

For Life: The Program

This program is gradual, progressive and, centering on areas of the body where amnesia has occurred. The first exercises will train you in sensitivity and control of muscles in the middle of your body. This is your center of gravity. The next deal with the periphery of your body: legs, arms and neck. The final one focuses on breathing and movement. This is a teaching method that involves a student to learn to move in slow, precise ways

Different movements change our muscular system by changing your central nervous system. This next part will tell you how to get maximum benefit from these new movements.

1. **Learn the nature of sensory-motor amnesia, how it occurs in your brain and where it occurs in your body:** Understand your brain and body are affected by stress and trauma. The initial effect from these movement patterns will feel like magic as your body relaxes and regains it suppleness. But, the real magic is in learning how to maintain this suppleness. Understand your body better. The more you understand your body the more you will discover about yourself. Every function you perform is controlled by your brain.
2. **Your primary task is to focus your attention on the internal sensations of movement.** As you perform concentrate on

Page39

developing a careful sensory awareness and maintain control over them. Each movement is described, then following is described for sensing so you know what to look for and how it should feel.

3. **Wear loose clothing and get yourself a yoga mat.** A mat provides a comfortable clean place to lie on. It offers you support. This allows you to be more precise I your movements. You will be loosening constricted muscles. You are not supposed to be working up a sweat. You will need to concentrate on the movement patterns and how they feel inside. Perceive the movements through feeling not by through your eyes. In other words, you need no mirrors. Wear, dance clothes or yoga pants etc. You need to be free of restricting clothes. If you have a recorder, record the lessons and they will always be handy.

4. **Always move slowly:** Moving slowly gives your brain a chance to notice what is happening in your body. The slower you move, the more you will perceive. Do not move onto the next movement until you are sure you know exactly what you are doing, and you can do it with ease and comfort. Repeat each lesson. Remember this is a progressive thing. The movements are programed at progressive levels. Master the exercises in each level.

5. **Always move gently with the least amount of effort:** This is so your brain can receive all the messages your body is sending it. It is better to feel you are doing too little than risk

too much. This undermines the work that these movements are doing.

6. **Do not force any movement:** This system will help you maintain sensitivity and control. No amount of effort will release the involuntary contractions in your body. Pushing against your muscles fails to release the hold of the amnesia. If you attempt to force, you will cause equal and opposite resistance, the muscle will contract tighter maybe even go into a spasm. Think of a knot, yanking on it just makes it tighter.

7. **Should never be painful:** These patterns are natural for the human body. If you perform them slowly and gently, they are completely harmless. Hurting yourself while exercising is unnecessary, harmful and no fun. Never mind the fact, it does not work. When muscles are tight, forcing movement makes the body tighten more. This causes avoidance of moving at all. Life is movement, so no one can avoid moving. The idea here is to move in the direction are, anatomically and neurologically designed. Yes, you might feel a little soreness when these muscles first begin to lengthen. This is normal. Once the muscles lengthen the soreness disappears. If you feel pain, move slowly and gently, never forcing the movements. You are trying to re-establish the natural movement of the human body. These movements are harmless if done properly.

8. **Be persistent, patient and positive:** These exercises change your body by teaching your

brain. Learning grows steadily and solidly. This is not a quick fix. It is genuine, lasting changes for your comfort, range of movement, posture and general functioning. Have positive expectations. The inability to move a muscle is known as Sensory Motor Amnesia

After you have mastered your sensory motor control maintenance comes into play. The learning stage requires patient attention. The maintenance stage is shorter and reinforces what you have learned. This means a short repetition of your basic movement patterns to remind the brain how the body should do them. These will be daily movements that should be done on awakening. Maintenance movements should not be thought of as exercises they are a natural way to prepare your body for the up-coming day. Also 5 minutes in the evening prepares you for a restful night's, sleep.

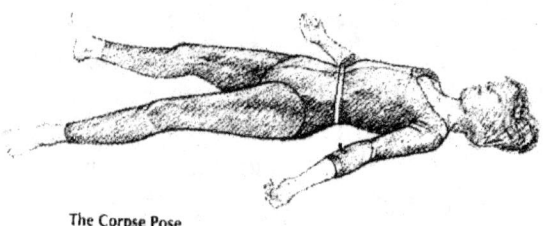

The Corpse Pose

SOMATICS

For all Stages of Life:

Chapter 3   General Uses!

Flexibility: Improves flexibility, range of motion and posture. Helps to manage pain. This is an essential part of everyday life. The more flexible the better off you are. Dancers need to stay flexible even though getting plenty of exercise through the dance. Flexibility corrects posture and improves range of movements, regardless of age. Stretching properly is an essential task in keeping your body ready for anything.

Posture: There are several benefits here. Stresses and strains on your spine can cause constriction of blood flow or nerves. Both cause serious issues on other parts of the body. Stresses on the spine can lead to poor posture. The human being has a central nervous system passes through and is protected by the spine. The spine keeps your body up-right. Looking after it is essential to your health and enjoyment of life.

Movement:

Fluid movement in all directions is the result of good posture and flexibility. The more movement the better. The more you move around the better the heart pumps. This ensures a plentiful supply of oxygen. A reduction in movement will result in doing less out of fear of injury. So, we do less and make the issue worse by having little motion.

Page43

Pain Management:

Pain is often the result of trauma. The muscles contract to deal with the injury. It may have been damaged by itself or reacting by protecting itself. You will be able to alleviate this pain by re-educating your muscles by learning how to control the muscles. Relaxing and stretching the muscles so the body can return to a stable position. Somatic movement is an excellent technique to target a wide range of ailments within the human body

Sciatica:

This nerve can become trapped, pinched or damaged. This results in a shooting pain down the leg. Learn how to stand correctly and control the muscles in your back. In this manner relaxing the sciatic nerve. This ensures it is relaxed and the pressure removed.

Hip, Knee and Leg Muscles:

These tightened muscles caused by either sitting much of the day or from running. Or doing things like dancing which is repetitive. The imbalance will cause imbalance to your joints and they will tighten due to the pressure being placed on them. Somatic exercises will relax the muscles and alleviate the pressure to your hips, knees and even your leg muscles.

Plantar Fasciitis:

Page44

This is pain and inflammation that people get in their feet. This is caused by tightening of the muscles in your legs and feet. This can be caused by years of bad habits. In dance it can be caused by years of poor technique. Replace your sub-conscious actions with a new way to move. You will benefit your health, posture and muscles.

TMJ Pain:

This pain occurs I the face, usually linked to stress. Many grind or clench the teeth. One needs to relax and re-train the muscles.

Here are other issues that can be relieved by Somatic movements.

Carpal Tunnel Syndrome
Tendonitis
Bursitis
Thoracic Outlet Syndrome
Chronic Headaches
Myo-facial Pain

Treatment sessions are short. It is highly effective and a long-term strategy.

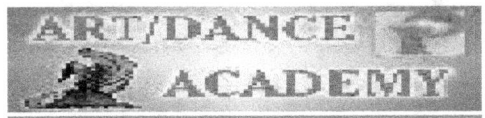

Later we will discuss more details on where, when and how.

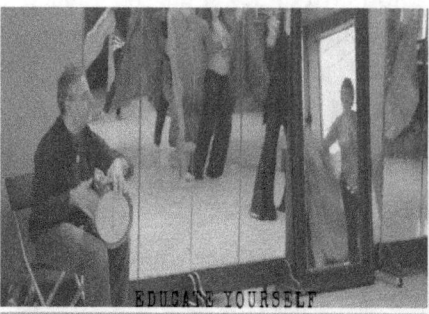
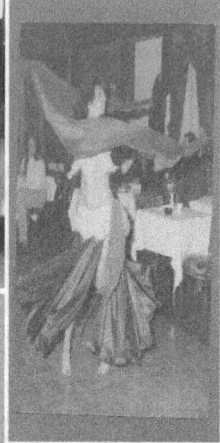
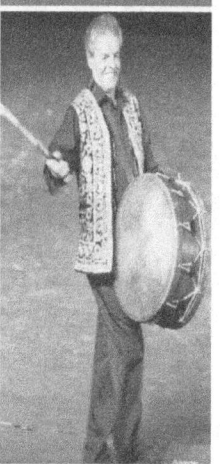
Morwenna & Walid Assaf

SOMATICS for

all Stages of Life:

Chapter 4   Where, When and How!

Somatic exercises will benefit everyone depending on the issues and injuries you have. It is the way of exercising and concept that is fundamental. You are doing three things in one movement. Remember, all movements must be done slowly and gently.

1. The first thing is: Because your muscle is to tighten your muscle more, this will remind the brain that the muscle is capable of different levels of contraction.
2. Next, you lengthen the muscle as much as possible. Then you release the muscle.
3. Finally, you relax the muscle as much as possible. Here the muscle will refocus its efforts into using the muscle correctly.

On Line or Local?

There may not be a class near you so on-line is where you go. There is an array of information on the internet. You need to assess what if what you are getting is valid. I am a believer of finding someone to at least talk to. As maybe you have found with dance teachers there is so much information, but you, have to, wade your way through it to find what is true and real. So be wary.

Reputation:
Confirm the references and reputation of the company. Look at the social media sites and see what people say. Assess the credibility of the firm before spending your, hard earned money.

Cost: This should always be a consideration. Look at all the possible and decide which place suits your needs, time and budget.

Recent for Treatment: Almost anyone can benefit from this treatment. Regular use of this treatment will improve your posture and reduce the stiffness It is unusual for anyone to realize they are in need if they are not in pain.

Understanding the Mind: The mind is more powerful than the body. The Somatic movements remind the brain of this.

Links to Yoga and Pilates: Yoga is great and very good for you. Am sure you can find, both of these classes in your locality. My preference being a dancer is Pilates. I used to have a reformer until I moved. Studied it for 3 years. Very beneficial. Yoga I personally did not like. I just wanted to get up and move. But that is a personal choice. Both excellent forms of movement. Somatic exercises are designed to take a minimal amount of time. The exercises are designed to stretch and relax muscles, no more!

Body Awareness: This exercise will help you to become more body aware. Lay on your back with mat with arms outspread. One hand up and the other face down. Roll your arms, both at the same time in opposite directions. 3 times/ Repeat 5-10 times. Keep the pace slow and coordinated.

Lower Back: This exercise can release and relax muscles plus help improve posture. Lie flat on your back legs extended. Twist right leg out, your lower back should arch. Hold for few seconds before twisting it inwards. The lower back should flatten out. Repeat with other leg. Do this several times then repeat with both legs at the same time. Be aware of how it feels. Repeat this with both legs 5 times. Note how the back feels.

Right and Left Back: This is an extension of the previous exercise. Bend knees a little. Roll legs together right and left 5-10 times. Then try 5-10 times with knees straight.

Spinal Freedom: Lie on back with knees bent and feet on the floor. Bring left leg to chest Use left hand to hold it in place. Place right hand behind head Lift head to left knee. Exhale while lifting head. Spine will lengthen. Hold a few seconds. Then lower letting back arch naturally. Repeat 3-5 times. Then do same with other leg etc.

Hamstrings: Sit on floor with legs in front. Bend right leg so foot is near crotch. Hold left leg. Bring head down towards knee. Repeat 3-5 times. Change legs.

Side Stretch: Standing. Feet in (2nd position parallel) under shoulders. Hands clasped behind head, elbows out. Breathe and lower body to one

Page49

side. Hold a few seconds. Repeat 3-5 times. Then repeat on other side. Then graduate to how you do it as a warm up in dance class. Remember to lift weight out of the body as you go over. This relieves pressure in the lungs.

Stretching the Thighs: Feet parallel under shoulders. Lift right leg in the back by stretching with the foot towards buttocks and gently stretch. Push pelvis slightly forward as leg pulls back to slightly relieve pressure on the knee. Repeat 3-5 times.

Neck & Shoulder: Lying down, extend legs. Lift arms straight up. Stretch one side further. Keep waist on the floor Hold for a few seconds then release. Do 2 more times. Switch and repeat on other side.

ELEMENTS!

Create A Space: The first thing you need to do is find a place to do your exercises. Clear enough space to lie down comfortably. Get that exercise mat I mentioned earlier. A bed can be used in a pinch. Have no outside interference. No tv, radio or music. Keep lighting subdued. Have cushions, yoga blocks or other props you may need close by

Clothing: Clothing does not have to be invested in. Just, make sure what you wear is comfortable and non-restricting.

Page 50

Breathing: Focus your breathing on exhaling as you start a movement and inhaling as you finish. Take long, deep slow breaths.

Speed: Slowly and smoothly is the way to go. Make sure you allow the time you need to allow your brain to focus. Focusing allows you to improve muscle coordination and your own awareness. Never push to the straining point. Explore your body, do not strain it. Only go as far as you can in any movement. Things will become easier and you then will achieve more. Your mobility and movement will improve but you have to stick to the exercises.

Muscles: The intention is to loosen the muscles. Focus on the muscles you are working on. When focusing on one muscle the others should be relaxed. That gets easier also with practice. You will even gain more control over your muscles as you go along. The more options you open will give you better quality of life. You will gain flexibility, better posture and broader movement.

Visualization: Visualize the movements before you start. This is the first step in creating a new behavioral pattern. Sounds like a dance class huh? Remembering learning new choreography or combinations.

Appreciation: Every movement has a noticeable benefit There for it is necessary to pause after each exercise. You want to absorb the feelings. Practice regularly, at least 4 or 5 times a week. This over and above your daily short sessions morning/evenings. The effects are cumulative, and you will quickly see the effects of the work you do.

USES FOR SOMATIC MOVEMENT

IMPROVEMENT

Simple somatic movements restore movement in painful muscles and improves flexibility and posture which is linked to re-programming your brain. The principle is based on the fact the body should be healed from the inside out. So, the brain relearns how to use the muscles properly. It is an option for anyone who suffers from decreased mobility, flexibility or bad posture. Regardless of your age or lifestyle you can benefit. Results will not be instant but given time you will see results.

It is all about rebalancing your body You work in every muscle individually. You are in control. You are the best person to teach yourself. You know which parts hurt or are limited. Focus and become self-aware. Somatic exercises take away bad habits. Your brain then becomes aware of how the muscle can be used. It removes the tension from the muscle and returns it to its original use and position. Your posture will improve almost instantly. You will stand taller and move better. Take the time to concentrate on posture, movement and flexibility. You have, to repeat it enough for it to be natural and automatic. Patience and practice will give you a lifetime of good posture, flexibility and freedom in movement. This is truly a step forward. This is also a preventative measure. It takes a little effort but can be done.

PAIN MANAGEMENT

Pain is the way of telling you that something in the body is wrong. This needs to be processed effectively. Your brain remembers the pain because it happens every time you do a certain thing in a certain way. You need to make a conscious effort not to fall into bad habits. The damaged part will stay damaged. Usually a muscle contracts to protect the injured area. This adds additional pain or tension and becomes locked into position. This can allow the area to heal. You can do something about this frozen muscle once the healing is complete.

You need to allow the body to completely relax and stretch will relieve the pressure on the muscle. This will allow the body to return to the pre-injury state of pain. The injury is gone. It is a natural form of healing. No herbs, no medicine. Through small movements the brain learns to re-control the muscles and return to former flexibility. Medicine only masks the symptoms. Somatic movement is long term healing.

Shallow Pain: Also called superficial pain. This is referring to a cut or a burn on the skin. These movements will not help this or hurt.

Deep Pain: Is usually a dull ache that will gradually wear you down. There can be sharp twinges doing specific movements. These are the

Page 53

movement we as humans try very hard not to make. This type of injury will need correcting via somatic movements to ensure that you use the muscles correctly. Regular painkillers and anti-inflammatories plus heat and cold have two issues.

1. <u>**1.**</u> Masking the pain helps you feel better but now you do not know your limits. So, you may overdo. This may cause more harm as you try to speed your recovery.
2. <u>**2.**</u> The other muscles that are protecting may remain contracted. Then you also lose muscle. Both contribute to limiting movement in the future and you risk long term pain.

Somatic movements can help with this scenario. Training your muscles to work properly and building the muscle up again. They will be taught to relax and stretch at your command.

ADVANTAGES AND DISADVANTAGES

As with everything in life there are pros and cons. You need to be aware of. These exercises are natural this ensures there is no risk to you.

ADVANTAGES: This is a method for treating aches and pains.

Time = Ten minutes is all you need. You can choose to do some exercises, stop and continue later. You can vastly improve your movement and flexibility through several (five minute) slots during the day. This makes it physically possible for anyone.

Page 54

Effectiveness = This form of exercises produces results quickly. So, with 10 or 12 directed sessions you will be well on your way. You will learn to understand the theory and learn to listen to your own body. From there you set up your exercises to your own needs. Listen to your body and never force anything.

Movement = Completing somatic exercises will release muscles that have been held and frozen for weeks, months or years. Your brain will allow you to relax your muscles, so you can move a specific joint in a way you might never have before. This will allow you to be more flexible and have a whole new way of moving properly the way the joints and muscles are intended.

Mobility = The more movement you gain, the more mobility you will gain without pain. You can achieve your goals to continue dancing, running or whatever. As pain lessens and joints become more flexible everything becomes much easier. Plus, your energy level will be boosted as the pain leaves.

Pain Relief = Living in pain is no fun. Pain seems to take over your life, it is hard to focus when everything hurts. You can throw away those prescriptions that can become addictive and can add to tiredness. The impossible now seems possible. Every time you repeat an exercise you are educating your brain, relaxing the muscles, and removing the pressure on your joints and other parts of your body. Pain pills will be needed less.

Page 55

Ease = These exercises can be performed almost anywhere. A mat can help but not a necessity. Carpeting can be fine. Clothes can be anything you are comfortable in.

Support = There is support and advice on line. Enlist the support of your family and friends. Anyone can do these exercises. They are easy and can be done by anyone. You need to be motivated to start and complete each and every exercise you undertake. Use these exercises along with your dance program. If you teach, you can add them to your warm up or cool down. (More on this later).

Connecting to the Body = You need to treat the body as a whole just as you do in your dance class. Not just the individual issues you have with it. Connect your mind and body. Develop an understanding of your body and mind. How do they relate to each other? This understanding will make it possible for you to achieve things you previously always thought impossible. Understand where your issues are and take the appropriate steps to fix them. That is what a good a good dance teacher or exercise practitioner is for. You deserve a balanced approach to life.

Muscle Control = Every somatic movement needs you to focus on specific muscles. You need to keep your focus on how it feels. What happens as you move, before, during and after each movement. Undertake this new challenge in a safe and knowledgeable way. Allow your body to dance and be up to the challenge. If you do not dance, then at least feel more comfortable with the improved posture and no pain. Your body deserves to live up to the challenge of life.

Injuries = Establish a regular pattern of movements to increase your body control. This ensures balanced muscles and that they are not contracting when you do not want them to or need to. Your muscles will be stronger and better able to adapt. You are less likely to become injured. In any form of exercise or dance technique is important for these reasons.

Improved Concentration = Although sessions are short you need to be completely in control of your focus. Be focused, at all times. This will help improve your concentration over all. This can help you learn faster. Important to all phases of life. If you are a dancer, you need to be in the moment.

DISADVANTAGES: Follow the exercises and perform as directed. Follow the guidelines.

Forcing the Movement = This is the first thing not to do. Every movement should be slow. You must learn to focus on how your body is reacting. Gradually stretch and improve movements, flexibility and posture while decreasing pain. Once you start experiencing some results, yea, you know it is working. Do not push harder or quicker for more results. This does not work!

Lack of Knowledge = A lack of understanding comes usually from not paying attention to your instructor or jumping the gun and assuming you know it. Lack of knowledge can be dangerous.

Page57

Remember a little education is worse than none. Pay attention. Go slowly. Learn all you can.

Too Fast, Too Soon = It is possible to force your body to do too much. This damages the benefits. Overdoing can cause adverse effect on other muscles, not the one you are working on. Retraining is the beginning. Just as you perform your exercises slowly also add new exercises slowly to increase your fitness and general well-being.

Newness of Treatment = There may be things not yet discovered about this form of treatment. We are in infancy here. Be open and keep abreast of things. This movement form is slowly becoming mainstream. These movements are designed to open up the mind. And use your own ability to improve movement and improve mobility, posture, flexibility and more.

Common Ailments That Can Benefit:

Arthritis-Painful inflammation of the joints.

Balance Problems-Unsteadiness when standing, walking or any kind of moving.

Dizziness-Altered sense of balance and place, lightheaded, feeling faint or as if head is spinning.

Frequent Urination-The need to urinate more often than is normal.

Obesity-The condition of being grossly fat or overweight. 30 lbs. overweight.

Sciatica-Pain affecting the back, hip or outer side of the leg. Caused my compression of a spinal nerve root in the lower back.

Tendinitis-A condition in which the tissue connecting muscle and bone becomes inflamed.

Uneven Leg Length-It is not the length of the leg bones that is causing uneven length. It is most likely the muscles in your waist and hips.

Whiplash-Injury caused by a severe jerk of the head that causes injury.

Low Self-Esteem-A person who feels unworthy, incapable and incompetent.

Somatic movements and exercises will open your mind. Explore the capabilities of your mind and body. Allow yourself to live a full life and be vital in all aspects.

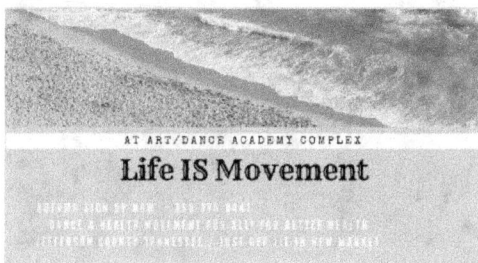

AT ART/DANCE ACADEMY COMPLEX
Life IS Movement

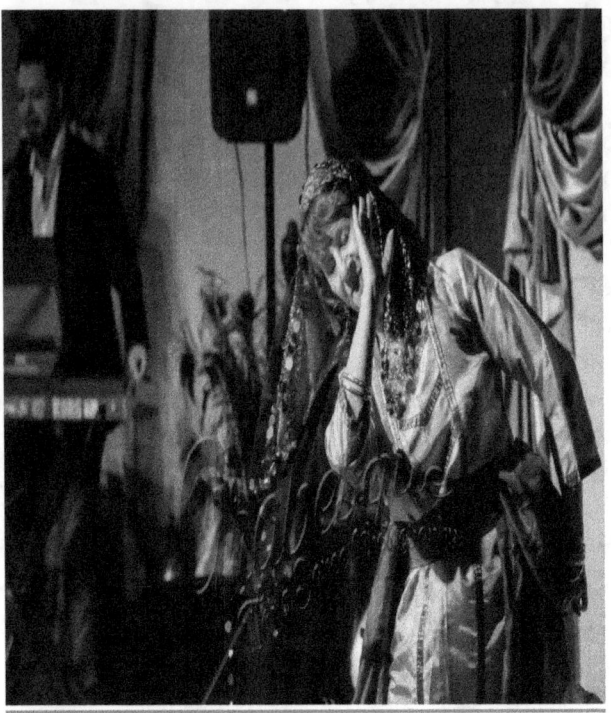

**Keep Moving – Morwenna & Fadi el Saadi
Lexington KY**

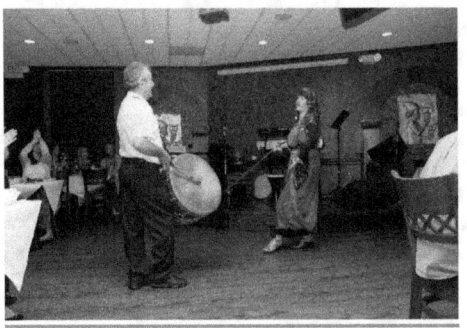

**Walid and Morwenna Assaf
Al Borz, Del Mar, CA**

Life IS Movement

PART 2

UNITY YOGA

Definition of Yoga means unity. Unity means a blend of mind and body.

Eight Reasons to Do Yoga

1. Lowers Stress and improves mood.
2. Boosts confidence.
3. Lowers risk of injury.
4. Helps you lose weight.
5. Increases flexibility.
6. Improves muscle tone and strength.
7. Benefits breathing and lowers blood pressure.
8. Improves posture

Youth Thru Yoga: Yoga poses stretch the muscles and increase range of motion. Not aerobic but as good for improving health. Increases range of motion, improves flexibility, builds muscle strength, perfects posture and prevents cartilage break down. Protects, your spine. Gives you better bone health. Increases blood flow. Drains lymph nodes and boost immunity. Helps control mind, body and soul. Brings together physical and mental disciplines for peace. Helps with stress and anxiety. Keeps one relaxed.

This is a form of gentle Yoga that anyone can do. What you do with it from here is up to you. All you need is you and a positive mind set.

Wear loose non-binding clothes.
If this is your bag, here it is. Works on Core for
Strength. Stretch to Increase Your Flexibility.
Balance for Stability. Flow- Reduces Stress.

When students first begin a yoga practice, perhaps
to reduce stress, get in shape, get stronger or maybe
just to accompany a friend, they will often place the
largest percentage of their attention on the poses
they are trying to do. This keeps the practice safe
and as we learn the postural integration. Our body-
based experience becomes more fulfilled, healthy
and more fun. Eventually, with skilled guidance one
becomes more interested not on the outer forms but
on the inner feelings that yoga can offer as well.
Pay attention the breath, the changes in the
emotional body. Recognize the mind as well as
thoughts, these are all part of yoga. It is a joining of
heart. Mind and body which provides health
benefits beyond just being strong and flexible.
The word, health is derived from an old English
word meaning "whole". Yoga re-establishes this
natural wholeness.

A morning practice can set you up for a day of
grace, authenticity, mindfulness and a positive
outcome. Can carry through a stressful workday.

With Yoga you can regulate your sleep patterns and
balance your hormones. Your body gets accustomed
to getting up and moving at the same time every
day. You will feel more energize and alert. Pay
attention to your breathing, this has a positive on the
endocrine system. The endocrine system uses
glands and hormones to help keep you balanced.

Certain poses increase melatonin. This helps you sleep better. That feeling of confusion or brain fog starts to disappear.

Boosting your metabolism by warming up your digestive system and helps nutrients move through your system more easily. This causes carbs and fats to metabolize more quickly. Even eases out aches and pains. More energy, more balance and a more restful sleep.

Stretching prevents injury and achiness throughout the day. Yoga lengthens and stretches tight bodies for all the day's movement. Yoga increases flexibility in the spine and encourages better posture. This sets our muscle memory for standing taller and walking and moving easier as the day progresses. This encourages good health for the entire day.

Consistent Routine:
Exercise regularly, at least 3x per week. This encourages you to stick with it. Know it is tough, to fit a fifteen – thirty-minute slot in our busy day and things do come up. Do it first thing in the morning with whatever time you have. Get it all done before you do anything else. You will feel good and feel good all day. Be disciplined and bring increase your mental strength in other areas of your life.

Here is How:
1. Specify a particular time. Practice Yoga or any form of exercise at a fixed time. Refresh your mind and release any stress. Fix a time, it is the best way to be consistent.

Page63

2. Choose a place that is where you will not be disturbed, a private corner will do. You need time for self, concentration and dedication.
3. Practice before you eat. Or wait 2-3 hours after eating.
4. Start easy as you are a beginner. Do easy poses and some stretching. Do not, risk straining your muscles. Be gentle it is not a heavy workout. Do not do it fast and do not take breaks in between.
5. Set the mood- Do it with a smile. Find inner peace. Dim the lights, put on soft music that will keep you motivated. Enjoy!
6. After you feel comfortable with what you are doing, try different poses and get more benefits.

Everything is useless unless you keep doing it. Make it a part of your daily habit.

If you have a medical situation check with your health care professional before starting.
Modify postures. If too tough modify Figure out what works for you. A feeling, yes but pain no. Start slowly and make sure you understand the alignment of the postures.

When you are ready to increase the intensity, try this: 1. Hold posture for longer and longer periods of time. 2. Slowly build up with more advanced and harder postures. 3. Go straight from one pose to another with no break. This is called flow.

Choose postures that look like you can do them. Start on the floor. Standing poses are harder and require more strength and balance.

Always practice between 15 and 90 minutes and repeat 3-6 times per week. Practicing more frequently with shorter times will yield greater will yield greater results. Wear comfortable clothes. Not something that restricts movement.

Remember workout on an empty stomach. Drink small amounts of water before starting. Do not drink during practice time if possible.

Now plan your time and get to it. Enjoy and do what you can with confidence. Enjoy!

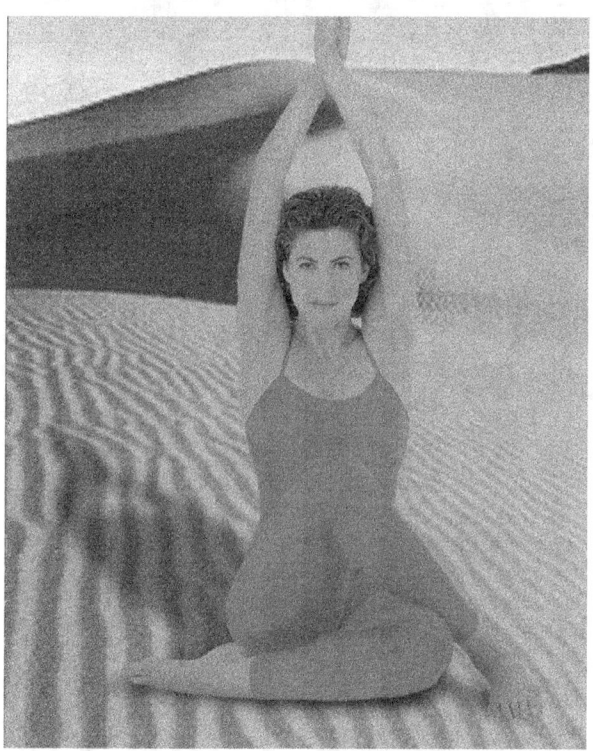

Page65

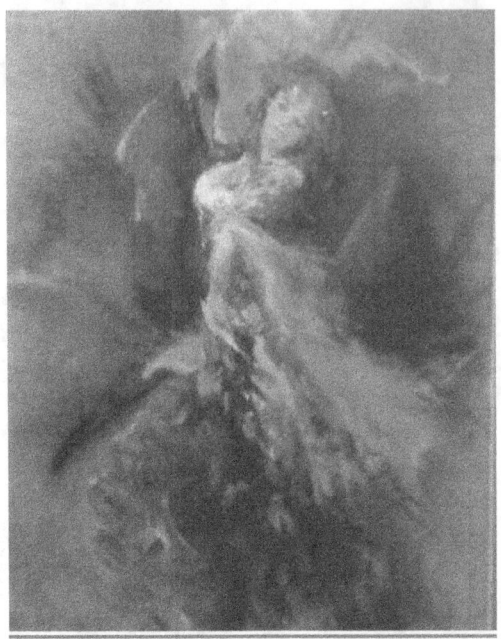

Morwenna Assaf Painting

byElisabeth Clark, Boston MA

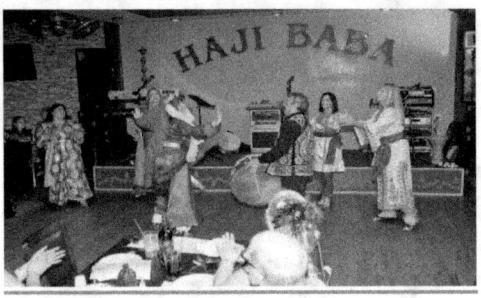

Morwenna and Walid with Raks el Anwar

Haji Baba, San Diego, CA

Life IS Movement

PART 3

PETITE PILATES

Easy Routines For All Ages

1. **Improve flexibility.**
2. **Strengthen and tone muscles.**
3. **Reduce stress.**
4. **Look and feel younger.**
5. **5 Eliminate aches and pains.**

Joseph Pilates was the founder of the Pilates method of exercise. He started by trying to strengthen his own body. You do not need weights or machinery to get or stay fit. You need regular functional exercise like stretching and flexing muscles, balancing and using your own body weight as resistance. Until fairly recently, it was one of the world's best kept secrets for getting and keeping strong and supple. Now, it is popular everywhere and people all over the world are enjoying its benefits.

Pilates is a unique form of simple, precise and affective exercises. It is gentle on the body but offers amazing benefits-focusing as it does on deep the deep muscles responsible for your body's core strength and stability. The exercises require a mental focus that helps you develop a greater understanding of how the body works. When you understand this, you can make it work more efficiently. In due time the correct movements will become automatic and you will sit, stand and move well all through the day.

Page67

The main aim is to improve posture by strengthening the stabilizing muscles of the torso. Your posture has a profound affect on your well-being. Imbalances in the spine can cause serious injury and lead to early aging. Start by leaving your preconceptions behind and be patient. Understand the new principles and allow your mind and body to adjust. Pilates is suitable for all levels of fitness at any age and is great for those with back pain or injury to the spine.

Here are some plus points in Pilates. 1. Better posture and improved coordination. 2. Ability to move well and freely. 3. Improved mental focus. 4. Automatic use of correct, efficient body movements and prevents strains and pains. 5. Increased muscular strength and flexibility. 6. Good fitness level and muscle tone. 7. Firm, flattened abdominal muscles. 8. A body that looks and feels younger.

In this day, and age, we are sedentary people who sit at desks to work all day. Before the coming of computers and yes typewriters we were all more active and out bodies had to work harder. We walked to work, rode a bike or took a bus or train. Today we just get in our car. Most of us have sedentary jobs and hectic lifestyles. We live with increasing amounts of stress. Excessive, amounts of stress, combined with long periods of physical inactivity can have a very bad effect on your health and well-being.

A sedentary lifestyle can result in muscles that are weak. Weak muscles can lead to poor posture, ill health, organ related diseases like heart disease and respiratory problems. Too often these things are put down to the result of increasing age, but this is wrong, and avoidable. Increased

Page 68

stress levels can lead to tight, aching muscles and untold strain on internal organs.

Pilates fits a busy lifestyle. It is not expensive. Does not require a lot of space. It can be done at home. Movements are slow and controlled. This minimizes the possibility of injury. So, all ages and all levels of fitness can do it. It includes deep breathing helps to reduce stress and calms the body and mind. Improve your core stability and you will maintain good posture, improved balance and have coordinated youthful movements.

The exercises are based on standing, lying, kneeling or sitting. You learn the poses and then they can be adapted for personal use. This workout takes 15-20 minutes and will leave you feeling stretched, energized and alive! Practice it regularly, at least, 2 or 3 times a week. You will achieve a flatter stomach, a better alignment, more elegant posture and increased strength and flexibility. In time, your body will look longer and leaner.

You do not need any special clothing or equipment. Just choose clothes that allow you to move freely. An exercise mat with a nonslip surface is useful to protect you from a hard, cold floor. It helps keep your feet and hands in position. You might want a cushion or towel for certain exercise.

A NUETRAL SPINE:

People come on lots of different shapes and sizes, but the basic design of the skeleton is the same for everyone and its alignment is the key to good posture. For most people, backache and most postural problems stem from the way they move. How we sit and stand, as well as lift and carry heavy items affects the body alignment. Postural changes can occur during pregnancy and giving birth. Even

overcoming an injury can have long-term effects on posture. One needs to remain supple and maintain good joint mobility, good pelvic and shoulder alignment with strong lengthened muscles. Pilates focuses on these elements to give you a well-aligned and well-balanced posture.

GOOD BREATHING:

In everyday life we take breathing for granted. We all know we have to breathe to stay alive, but most of us are unaware of the importance of breathing correctly. In Pilates you breathe by slowly expanding and contracting your lungs-moving only your ribcage and keeping the rest of the body still. You need to expand your ribcage sideways and backwards on the inhale and close the ribcage, engage the pelvic floor muscles and pull the navel in and up as you exhale. This movement of the ribcage activates the muscles between the ribs and those around the spine at the back of your ribcage. You need to choose a peaceful, warm place to practice so you can focus on your breathing in comfort.

ABOUT BODY AWARENESS:

It is important to warm up the body before you move on to mat work. Tis helps to prepare you mentally and physically for more strenuous exercises. Time spent correcting your posture and focusing on breathing improves technique and mental focus. Make sure your head and pelvis are correctly aligned.

WORKING YOUR CORE MUSLCES:

Page 70

The core muscles of your torso are responsible for keeping the spine in neutral alignment Concentrate on mobilizing and maintaining these core muscles is important. Good spinal alignment helps keep the heaviest parts of the body in balance. This includes pelvis, ribcage and head. Good balance minimizes stress on the joints. If there is any imbalance it will affect your posture, which can lead to pain and injury. Putting your head forward will shorten the neck muscles. It creates tightness in your shoulders and can cause headaches. Round your shoulders, the front of your ribcage sinks then the chest muscles tighten. This reduces mobility of muscles and restricts space for vital organs.

ABOUT BACK LENGTHENING AND STRENTGHENING:

This will improve your shoulder alignment for good posture and increase flexibility in the spine. The muscles of the back and front of your torso work together to stabilize your body, keeping bones and muscles in balance. While you are exercising your stomach you are also working your back muscles. The opposite is true. This will give you a more defined shape, especially around the bra line. It will strengthen the muscles that run along the spine which will improve shoulder alignment and make your back more flexible. The muscles in your back play a monumental part in good posture. We tend to spend so much time sitting and driving with our abdominal muscles disengaged. So, these muscles become weak and create unbalanced posture.

Art / Dance Academy Complex

www.danceranddrummer.com

STAYING STRONG

ABOUT EXERCISING ON ALL FOURS:

Exercises done kneeling on all fours are designed to improve mobility of the spine plus strengthen and the abdominal and back muscles plus generally improve posture. This may feel uncomfortable. If so give yourself more padding by placing a thin cushion or towel under your knees. If wrists feel stiff place palms on small, soft foam balls. This relieves the pressure. The aim is to stretch to improve flexibility of the spine, lengthen the back muscles and improve awareness of correct breathing, neutral spine and abdominal stability.

ABOUT SEATED EXERCISES:

Keeping your spine neutral while doing seated exercises is challenging. They provide a demanding and exciting extension to movements. Lengthy sitting encourages bad posture. The invention of the chair does us no favors. Sitting so much is detrimental to our back health. As children we are so much more flexible. We spent time crawling, playing and sitting on the floor. But, as adults we sit in chairs. The result causes hamstrings and back muscles to weaken and shorten. Seated Pilates exercises are practiced in good postural alignment with legs outstretched. As you progress this gets easier as you develop strong and lengthen muscles. Concentrate on lengthening hamstrings. Postural problems often start from bad sitting habits. Seated exercises help to improve your seated posture, an improvement that you should continue throughout the day.

ABOUT DEEP ABDOMINAL EXERCISES:

These exercises provide a strong challenge for the abdominal muscles. Make sure your breathing technique is strong and your control of the spine is too. While exercises lying on your back look easy, they can be deceptive. The movements require both muscular control and strength. Do not try to ne over ambitious, especially in the beginning. Do fewer repetitions and focus on joint alignment and breathing. They will improve your core muscular strength hand help streamline your body. This will give you a longer, leaner look. Lying on your back is the most restful position for your spine and an easy way to find neutral spine. The neck and shoulder area is where many people hold stress especially when tired, worried or have jobs that involve sitting for long periods. This will cause weak, tight muscles in shoulders, headaches and back pain. Releasing tension form the neck and shoulders helps improve your posture and relieves everyday aches and pains.

ABOUT A FAST TRACK WORKOUT:

This is where you bring isolated exercises together to form a flowing routine. It also helps refine the technique. Every time you practice Pilates you are gently educating your body. Moving away from old habits and developing a personal body awareness. Making it flow will add another dimension to the way you challenge your body. It links in a flowing succession in different positions to take you to a new level. Fast Track should take about 15 minutes and be easy to fit into any busy schedule. It can be performed any time during the day.

The workout starts standing to warm-up. Always check posture before starting. Make sure ankles, knees and his are in alignment and your weight is evenly distributed. Pelvis should be in neutral. Align neck and shoulders. Draw chin in so your neck is lengthening and have a feeling that you are lifting from the top of the head. Practice deep breathing before you begin. Remember to breathe through each movement and keep the exercises gently flowing.

WHEN YOU REACH A NEW LEVEL:

The more advanced level of Pilates exercises, require and build increased strength, mobility and flexibility. Practicing Pilates gives you gives you a heightened awareness of your body and its needs. This allows you to educate the muscles in a controlled and progressive way. It is considered the thinking person's exercise. Try Pilates to test your body awareness.

PILATES FOR HEALING:

PREVENTING BACK PAIN:

Back pain especially in the lower back is often caused by bad posture. Sitting for long periods, repeated bending, heavy lifting, and standing or lying in awkward positions can all create back pain. You can take steps to help yourself by improving your posture when lifting, sitting and carrying.

1. Lift items correctly,
2. Carry bags in alignment

RELIEVING LOWER BACK TENSION:

Tight hamstrings in the legs can cause hip-joint problems, this leads to lower back pain. You need to stretch the hamstrings and lengthen the spine, hips and calves.

RELIEVING UPPER BACK TENSION:

The aim here is to relieve the pain, improve flexibility in the upper back and neck. This area is where the movement of the spine is often restricted by weak, tight muscles.

RELIEVING SHOUDER AND NECK TENSION:

Open the chest and stretch across the front. If the pectoral muscles are tight it causes the shoulders to become rounded. Also relieve tight, sore neck muscles to get rid of headaches.

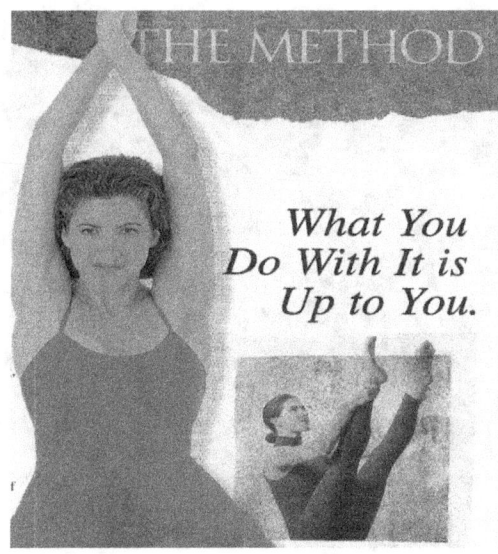

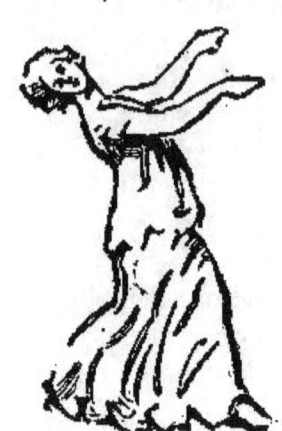 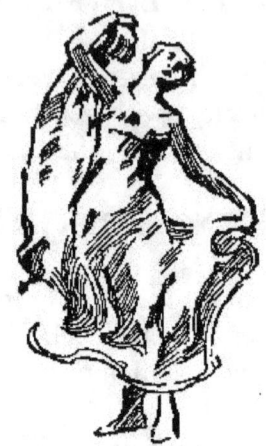

Lebanese prints of

Ancient Dancers

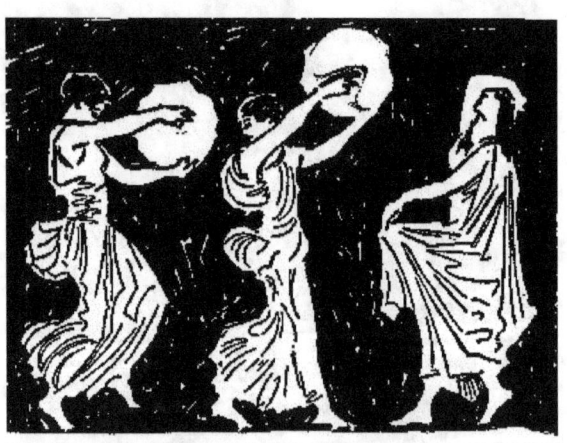

Life IS Movement

PART 4

BASIC BALLET BARRE

The Best Exercise for ALL Ages

Doing a Ballet Barre is the best system for conditioning. But not a place to start unless you were a trained dancer. As with all forms. Start slow and build. It is a system, developed over the centuries, whose goal is to strengthen the body while molding it into an ideal of grace and beauty. It can be fun, effective and when done with the proper technique, safe. It has the cardiovascular benefits of aerobic dance when done center floor with corresponding steps. It helps develop fluidity of movement and poise as no other form of exercise can. Also, you can look refined and graceful while doing it. The benefits are great too.

There are special aspects to ballet that need to be thought of. It is safe! Maybe safer than going to Zumba, Aerobics or an exercise class. A dancer's body is her instrument, so it must be protected at all costs. The exercises covered here are not just for those who want to do a series of dance exercises. It is used as a form of warm-up for any kind of activity or just as a form of exercise alone. Your body will thank you as it requires your body to be limber and to avoid strain and injury You will perform any activity with more control and finesse.

Basic Ballet Barre is by its very nature a built-in safety factor. You do not need to lie on the floor or sit at a machine or use weights. You are standing, bending, reaching and turning, all everyday natural movements. Your body is always under control. Control is the essence of ballet even at this basic level. It is this constant control, even while seemingly doing effortless movements that develops strength and endurance. At the same time, control prevents strain and injury. The fact that all the movement are natural to the human body. It brings grace to everyday movements. Dancers are not only graceful when they dance, they are graceful when they sit, stand and walk. Dancers can often be picked out in a crowd because of their poise. This is because it works the whole body - head, arms, legs, hips and torso. No one part is emphasized at the expense of another. The goal is appearance as well as movement and strength as a graceful unit. This can be learned. Basic Ballet Barre will make every day a natural habit of graceful movement.

Basic Ballet Barre is also remarkable at shaping your body. Ballet emphasizes long, lithe muscles. It creates them. Determination, along with regular work, can shape a less than perfect body into a body of perfection. The average woman can gain this look. Most women are not interested in bulky muscles, they want to look sleek, firm and toned.

There is nothing better than a Ballet Barre to gain this look, in todays' society. It is always good to have a body in proportion but if you are not tall and willowy do not think you cannot enjoy ballet. Some movements are best executed by short people and some by tall. We all have out thing. So, do not let height or body build keep you from the beauty of ballet. The exercises and movements of ballet are designed to look good; it is, after all, a visual art. Women look beautiful when doing ballet barre exercises. The movements are fluid. The music is delightful. The whole atmosphere Basic Ballet Barre is romantic. Who could ask for anything more. Try it and agree.

We talk about posture, but, really what is it? Ask yourself this question. Good, posture-what is it? The correct line of the body is called "alignment" in ballet. Correct posture is absolutely, crucial to get the most out of your Basic Ballet Barre. Correct posture in motion, is alignment. Do all exercises very slowly so you can concentrate on your posture with the correct placement of arms, legs, hips, head and torso. You need to stand like a dancer. Learning how to stand and hold yourself properly takes effort at first. Keep at it, it will become second nature. It is only by working in the correct positions that you will benefit by these exercises. You need to become conscious of every part of your body. These movements will make you develop an awareness. It should not be exaggerated.

POSTURE

Good posture—The correct line of the body in dance is called alignment. It is crucial if you want to get the most out of any exercise program. Ballet is simply put, correct posture in motion. Do all exercises very slowly, especially in the beginning. Concentrate on posture and correct placement of arms, legs, hips, head and torso. Almost all ballet exercises, begin the same way. You do not need perfection, but you do need to learn to stand and move like a dancer. Learning how to stand and move takes effort at first, but then becomes second nature. But it is only by learning the correct placement that you will experience the benefits of these exercises. You need to become conscious of every part of your body. These exercises will give you the awareness. Once the posture is automatic, the positions and movement will be done with ease and become graceful. They will then feel natural. You want to feel graceful, when working your hardest.

Page 79

FEET

Your feet need to be relaxed. Do not grab the floor with your toes. Most of the weight of your body should be resting on three (3) spots: Your heel, your little toe and your big toe. Like a tri-pod. Do not let your ankles roll in or out. Ankles out of alignment will throw the line of your whole body out of whack and could result in a strained muscle. Try putting a mirror in front of your feet. Check to see if your ankles are straight, the weight should be correctly distributed across the ball of each foot.

TURN-OUT

Feet can be slightly turned out or in parallel. In classical Ballet the feet are turned out. We can work at both 45degree turnout or perpendicular. The whole leg rotates from the hips. Do not try to exaggerate your turn-out. You will lose your alignment and even strain a muscle especially of the ankles and feet. Turn out your toes by rotating from the hips, only as far as is comfortable. Your body should never be stiff. Your ankles must be straight and your knees above your feet. In fact, over your 2nd and 3rd toes. Your body must be relaxed and free to move.

LEGS

If your posture is good and your feet are placed correctly, your legs will be placed properly. Before you start to move in any direction make sure your knees should be straight but not locked. Your knees should point in the same direction as the toes. Check this! You should feel the muscles of the thighs pulling up. There should be a slight tension but never stiffness in those muscles.

Page 80

TORSO

To get your torso into proper alignment, focus on rib-cage, tummy and backside. The backside is the tough one. The best way to correct this problem is to lift the rib cage by inhaling and expanding the chest and shoulders. Then, tighten the abdominal muscles right in the center of your ribs. Stand t a slight angle to the mirror and see the buttocks fall into perfect alignment. This also slims your waist. Always remember to pull up from the waist while keeping the shoulders down. Imagine a string attached to your breastbone that is pulling your chest up and slightly forward. This achieves an open lifted look and feeling.

ARMS AND HANDS

When you do your Basic Ballet exercises you will be using your arms and hands for balance and for grace. The main idea in the positioning of the arms is to achieve a graceful line. As for balance, using your arms in the correct positions can help steady you when doing certain movements. Your arms should be slightly curved, never completely straight. This is true of the hands too. To help achieve this look. Shake your hands a few times, then stop, your hands should them be relaxed. Understand that while arms and hands should be relaxed, they should never be limp. Shoulders should be pressed down, , no matter where the arms are

HEAD

The desirable look is that of a swan. Hold the head high, lengthening the line of the neck and holding the head high. Have the neck relaxed and do not stick chin out-keep it parallel to the floor.

Page 81

CHECK LIST

STARTING POSITION:

1. Feet: Feet with heels (1" apart) Toes turned out as far as is comfortable. Or feet parallel 1 or 2 inches apart.
2. Legs: Thigh muscles pulled up
3. Torso: Chest lifted from breast-bone, Stomach engaged, rear-end neutral.
4. Head: Neck long, chin forward but not stuck out.
5. Arms: Slightly curved at elbow and wrist. The hands a few inches in front of the thighs. Hands graceful and curved, palms facing each other. Shoulders down.

THE PLIE:

The plie is a basic ballet move. A plie involves bending the knees and lowering the torso while keeping the body straight. Sometimes done in 1st or 2nd position. Your bent knees should always remain over the foot. Upper body does not change as your knees bend. Head is high, chest lifted and back straight. This is an exercise that increases strength and flexibility in legs.

BREATHING:

Breathing while you do any form of exercise is very important. It affects the way look in the line of the body. But, breathing is not for looks only. When you breathe deeply, your spine is lengthened, and your waist slimmed down. Breathing makes enough oxygen to work the muscles. You must breathe deeply to exercise. Inhale through your nose and fill lungs completely with air. If you inhale when rising from a plie you will lighten the upper body and achieve better line and balance.

SOME OTHER THOUGHTS

THE FLOOR: The floor is not a landing pad, it is a spring board. In a plie the body goes down but really wants to stay up. You always have to shift weight for whatever you are doing. R-L or forward and back.

SUPPORT: At the barre you work on the basic form and technique. You need to have support a chair back is good. It is to support you, not bear your weight. Do not lean on it, just a light touch will do. Most exercises can also be done center floor.

A MIRROR: This is how you check to see if your hips are straight and your arms are correct. You need to make peace with the mirror. This fills the gap of what a step feels like and what it looks like. You make corrections here. Do not let it be a crutch. Do not become obsessed with looking in the mirror. Be realistic and do not let it get in your way.

MUSIC: Music and tempo are important. Plus, it makes everything more fun. Music also dictates the speed and emphasis of the exercise. It also helps you remember. You need to feel the rhythm of the movement.

CLOTHES: When it comes to exercise, anything goes. You only have yourself to please. The best

Page83

dance outfits though are tights or jazz pants and a form fitting top. I happen to love leg-warmers. So, I wear them all year. But they are especially useful for keeping calf and ankle muscles warm in the cooler months. For a leaner look, keep your attire all in one color and preferably a dark color.

HAIR: Tie it back in a ponytail or in a braid. Even a headband might keep it out of your face.

SHOES: You can exercise in bare feet. If you do decide to buy exercise shoes makes sure they are well fitted and the correct type. No, sneakers! Sneakers do not allow you to work your foot properly. You can buy traditional ballet shoes with a soft leather sole. Elastic comes with them and a good knowledgeable person on dance can tell you how to sew the elastic. It is easy. Break your shoes in before wearing. Just knead and twist them with your hands.

Now begin to dance and enjoy!

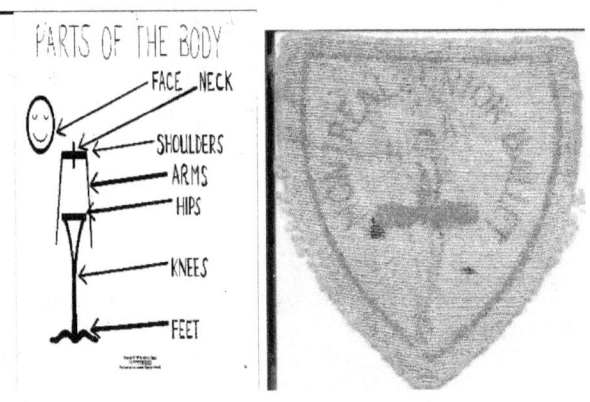

Life IS Movement

PART 5

RHYTHM REMEDY

Rhythm Remedy:- The skillful use of music and rhythm with musical elements promotes, maintains and restores mental, physical, physical, emotional and spiritual health. It is a non-verbal, creative with structural and emotional qualities. It treats depression and anxiety and other diseases. Effective, for all ages and abilities. Addresses a person's needs. Works with person through playing the rhythms and listening to music.

Rhythm helps to improve everything from speech to physical balance. Improves respiration, lowers blood pressure, reverses cardiac output, lowers heart rate and relaxes muscle tension. Rhythmic music may change brain function. Beats may encourage and alert concentrated thinking. Rhythm is fundamental in so many ways. Lasting gains in concentration and performance. Can reverse blood flow to the brain in the elderly.

For most people, music is an important part of daily life. Some rely on music to get them through the morning commute, while others turn up a favorite playlist to stay pumped during a workout. Many folks even have the stereo on when they're cooking a meal, taking a shower, or folding the laundry.

Modern music therapy aims, by the use, of music to improve <u>health</u> or functional outcomes in people. It typically involves regular meetings with a qualified music therapist and various combinations of music-related activities. In 'active therapy' the individual and therapist make music using an instrument or the voice; in 'passive therapy' the individual listens to music in a reflective mode. You don't have to be musical to take part. And, of course, you don't have to take part to engage with music.

Music is often linked to mood. A certain song can make us feel happy, sad, energetic, or relaxed. Because music can have such an impact on a person's mindset and well-being, it should come as no surprise that music therapy has been studied for use in managing numerous medical conditions.

All forms of music may have therapeutic effects, although music from one's own culture may be most effective. In Chinese medical theory, the five internal organ and meridian systems are believed to have corresponding musical tones, which are used to encourage healing.

Types of music differ in the types of neurological stimulation they evoke. For example, classical music has been found to cause comfort and relaxation while rock music may lead to discomfort. Music may achieve its therapeutic effects in part by elevating the pain threshold.

Music may be used with guided imagery to produce altered states of consciousness that help uncover hidden emotional responses and stimulate creative insights. Music may also be used in the classroom to aid in the development of reading and language skills. Receptive methods involve listening to and responding to live or recorded music. Discussion of their responses is believed to help people express themselves in socially accepted ways and to examine personal issues.

1. **AUTISM**: People who have autism often show an interest in and have a heightened response to music. This may aid in the teaching of verbal and non-verbal

communication skills. And it also helps to establish normal developmental processes.

2. **DEMENTIA**: In older adults with Alzheimer's, dementia, and other mental disorders, music therapy has been found to reduce aggressive or agitated behavior, reduce symptoms of dementia, improve mood, and improve co-operation with daily tasks, such as bathing. Music therapy may also decrease the risk of heart or brain diseases in elderly dementia patients.

3. **DEPRESSION**: Depression or depressive disorder is an illness that involves the body, mood, and thoughts. Depression is considered a mood disorder. Depression affects the way a person eats and sleeps, the way one feels about oneself, and the way one thinks about life situations. Unlike normal emotional experiences of sadness, loss, or passing mood states, depressive disorders are persistent and can significantly interfere with an individual's thoughts, behavior, mood, activity, and physical health.

There is evidence that music therapy may increase responsiveness to antidepressant medications. In elderly adults with depression, a home-based program of music therapy may have long-lasting effects. In depressed adult women, music therapy may lead to reductions in heart rate, respiratory rate, blood pressure, and depressed mood. Music therapy may also be beneficial in depression following total knee replacement surgery or in patients undergoing hemodialysis.

4. **INFANT DEVELOPMENT:** There is evidence that music played to the womb during late pregnancy may lead to children being more responsive to music after birth. Soothing music may help newborns be more relaxed and

Page 87

less agitated. Pre-term newborns exposed to music may have increased feeding rates, reduced days to discharge, increased weight gain, and increased tolerance of stimulation. They may also have reduced heart rates and a deeper sleep after therapy.

5. SLEEP QUALITY: Insomnia is difficulty in falling asleep, staying asleep, and waking up too early in the morning. It is a common health problem that can cause excessive daytime sleepiness and a lack of energy. Long-term insomnia can cause an individual to feel tired, depressed or irritable, have trouble paying attention, learning, and remembering, and not be able to perform fully on the job or at school. Severe insomnia can result in neurochemical (brain chemical) changes that may cause problems such as depression and anxiety, further complicating the insomnia.

In older adults, music may result in significantly better sleep quality as well as longer sleep duration, greater sleep efficiency, shorter time needed to fall asleep, less sleep disturbance, and less daytime dysfunction. There is also evidence of benefit in elementary-age children or stable preterm infants. Music therapy may also be as effective as chloral hydrate in inducing sleep or sedation in children undergoing EEG testing.

6. **SAFETY**: Just as certain music can help induce relaxation and peaceful states, other music may cause agitation. There is evidence that music that reflects the listener's personal preference is more likely to have desired effects. It is possible that music through headphones during medical procedures could interfere with the patient's cooperation with the procedures. Also, listening to music at

high volumes may damage the ears and lead to hearing loss.

The oldest musical instruments to have been found — flutes made from bird bone and mammoth ivory — are more than 42 thousand years old; and it has been argued that, by fostering social cohesion, music—from the Greek, 'the art of the muses'— could have helped our species outcompete the Neanderthals. Remember that next time you stand to the national anthem.

Music should not be used as the sole treatment for potentially dangerous medical or psychiatric conditions. Use is not recommended in those who do not like music therapy as this may result in agitation or stress.

Since then music is a pleasure, and virtue consists in rejoicing and loving and hating aright, there is clearly nothing which we are so much concerned to acquire and to cultivate as the power of forming right judgments, and of taking delight in good dispositions and noble actions. Rhythm and melody supply imitations of anger and gentleness, and also of courage and temperance, and of all the qualities contrary to these, and of the other qualities of character, which hardly fall short of the actual affections…

Does music therapy work? People ask me all the time, "How does music therapy work?" At first I start preparing an answer about its effectiveness. Quickly, though, it becomes clear they're asking a question that seems simple but is in fact just as complicated.

They want to know what happens during a session. Do you listen to recordings? Do you sing songs? If so, who does it? The client, or the therapist?

The answer is yes. The practice of music therapy represents a rich and varied set of traditions co-existing under one big tent.

Walking in rhythm is its own kind of music, and I believe it is a bad idea to walk while wearing headphones. They block you from experiencing the world. It is of course tempting to listen to your favorite tunes, especially since there is no better motivator than a walking beat. But if you use earbuds or, even worse, headphones that go over the ear, you are by definition not paying attention to the sounds around you. This is the same problem as distracted driving. One way to avoid the earbud problem is to buy a portable Bluetooth speaker, which people hang from their belts while they walk or run. Do not do this. Blasting your music so that others can hear it is antisocial. On your next walk sing your favorite songs.

Here's how to walk with music: The aboriginal peoples are wrapped up in both walking and singing. A big part of the story is the discovery that aboriginal singing is a kind of aural map—that the song and the land are one. "Music is a memory bank for finding one's way about the world." The author muses out loud about evolutionary biology and the nomadic origins of our species. Humans, it is concluded, we were built for walking. Be sure to bring something to write on when inspiration strikes. Think of the military who walk and sing patriotic songs.

Music therapy has a unique ability to reach people with dementia. In some cases, clients might be able to make music of their own, or perhaps only listen. Better yet, spend your walk writing songs of your own. The easiest way to start is by creating new lyrics to pre-existing melodies. Anyone can do this.

Then you have music psychotherapy, an alternative to the talking cure. Practitioners align themselves with any number of orientations, from psychoanalysis to humanistic psychology to CBT. Therapy happens in any number of ways, including improvisation, writing new lyrics to existing songs, you name it.

And if so, how? Music boosts levels of dopamine, a feel-good chemical messenger in the brain. Many people use music to power through a workout. Beyond distracting from discomfort, music triggers the release of opioid hormones that relieve physical and psychological pain. Forget the workout, just dance to the music. Dancing is the best exercise because it involves movement in all directions and engages the mind on multiple levels. Music also boosts the immune system, notably by increasing antibodies and decreasing stress hormones, which can depress the immune system. Techno and heavy metal aside, music lowers heart rate and blood pressure, and even reduces recovery time following a heart episode or surgery.

From a more psychological perspective, music therapy alleviates symptoms of anxiety and depression and improves social and occupational functioning. Aside from the biological benefits such as increased dopamine and decreased stress hormones, music can help us to recognize, express, and process complex or painful emotions. It elevates these emotions and gives them a sense of legitimacy, of order, beauty, and meaning. We hear a human voice and feel understood. As Taylor Swift put it, "People haven't always been there for me, but music always has."

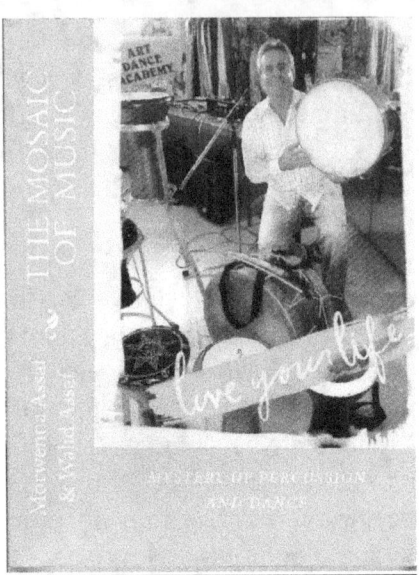

Walid Assaf and Mosaic of Music

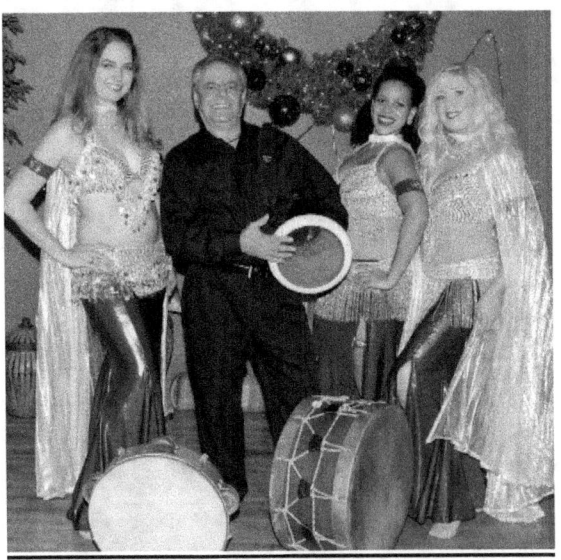

Walid and Dancers Knoxville TN

Life IS Movement

PART 6

NATURAL NUTRITION

NATURAL NUTRITION

Nutrition is supposed to help you not hurt you. So, you need to be careful of what you choose to eat. Food is a critical part of the wellness plan for all. The wrong food can cause pain, inflammation, being overweight and having low energy. Unfortunately, the typical diet eaten by most Americans supports ill health by consisting of all the wrong things including sugar, processed meats preservatives etc. A proper diet is anti-inflammatory and full of great nutrition. This relieves pain, inflammation and weight. We all have different needs. All of the former chapters are no help if you are not eating correctly for your body and needs.

Food is a double-edged sword that can both cause and reduce inflammation etc. You need the right mix for your body. What is good for one person is not necessarily good for another. Choose from good foods for better health and welfare.

There are seven areas of food to avoid if you have pain and inflammation. Most infections are caused by inflammation. Here is a list by Dr Mark Wiley.

1. **Animal Milk Products** – milk, cream, cheese, cottage cheese, yogurt and ice cream.
2. **Hydrogenated Oils** – Non -dairy creamer, crackers, cookies, chips and snack bars.

3. **Nitrates** – Hot dogs, cold cuts, pepperoni, sausage, bacon and liverwurst.
4. **Processed Sugar** – Candy, soda, bread, bottled fruit juice, cookies and snack bars.
5. **Nightshades** – Potatoes, peppers, tomatoes, eggplant and paprika.
6. **Convenience Food** – French fries, onion rings, loaded bake potatoes, fatty burgers, Mexican food, pizza, calzones and stromboli.
7. **Processed White Flour Products** – Flour, bread, pasta, pizza, crackers, pretzels and donuts.

As you can see this is the sample of most Americans diet. We are also the most overweight and pain suffering people in the world. These ingredients are found in every snack and even so-called healthy foods. Do not believe marketing. Read the labels. By eating these foods, you are increasing the possibility of inflammation and the longevity of the pain. You are adding to your own pain.

Foods That Reduce Pain and Inflammation:-

Food is the substance of life along with air and water.

Here is the list of best-known foods to work with you. These should be part of everyone's balanced wholesome foods.

A diet high in fiber and whole foods, low in preservatives and unhealthy fats can help you reduce your feeling of not being up to par. These foods not only reduce pain and inflammation but also support proper nerve function and bone health.

Page94

1. **General Foods:-** Wild Alaskan Salmon 2. Fresh whole fruits 3. Bright colored vegetables 4. Green or white tea 5. Purified and distilled water. 6. Healthy Oils- Olive, Flax, Hemp, Safflower, Hazelnut or Coconut 7. Organic Beef or Poultry 8. Nuts, legumes and seeds 9. Dark leafy green vegetables. 10. Organic Oatmeal 11. Spices: Turmeric, ginger, cloves, garlic, onion, coriander and mustard seed.
2. **Green Tea**: - Full of vitamin C and E. Two to Four cups recommended.
3. **Mushrooms**: - Boost immunity. - Six reasons mushrooms are so healthy for you

A. Excellent dietary staple to boost health

B. They contain 30% of high-quality proteins and all nine essential amino acids.

C. The fat is them is unsaturated and in very low levels.

D. They contain more mineral salts than most meat and nearly double that of vegetables.

E. High in phosphorous, potassium and contain calcium, magnesium, aluminum, zinc and copper plus vitamins B1, 2, 3 and 9.

F. Useful for the treatment of diseases caused by low immunity like rheumatoid arthritis, HIV, lupus, connective tissue disease, hypertension, heart disease, diabetes, kidney problems, viral infections, malnourishment, cancers, tumors and convulsions.

Add them to your meals.

4. **Turmeric:** Actually, an Indian cornerstone of Ayurvedic medicine. It is the component of curcumin in them that makes them so beneficial Curcumin reduces inflammation naturally unlike aspirin or ibuprofen. Treats arthritis, sports injuries, IBS, Crohn's disease, various autoimmune diseases and research is being done for those suffering from asthma. Is also an antioxidant and used in treating wounds, digestive disorders, liver issues, prevention of cancer and helps reduce side-effects of cancer treatment, chemo-therapy.

5. **Water Hydrates Also Flushes Toxins: -** Drink ample amount of water every day. A sluggish digestive system, liver and kidneys contribute to and trigger pain processes. The mere consumption of water can help restore the body to its natural state. It clears toxins, cleanses the colon, flushes liver and kidneys and empties bowels. Toxins get trapped in muscle tissue and joints. This creates pain and swelling. Flush them out. A slow metabolism and elimination can lead up to a build-up of toxins in the blood. This can manifest into headaches, fibromyalgia and arthritis pain.

6. **Eating And Weight Loss: -** We live on food, water, oxygen and sunlight. On a basic level fuel is fuel. This gives us energy. It nourishes the body, cells, organs, brain and every tissue.

   When trying or needing to lose weight keep these five points in mind.

1. Stop looking at food in terms of deconstructed parts. This only tells you part of the story and adds to the confusion and stress. So, no more, protein, fat etc.

2. Start looking at food in global terms of how ingredients or products interact with other food and how your body handles it.

3. What is relevant is what happens to it when it reaches your digestive track. How quickly does it digest? How rapidly the food breaks down into sugar? How fast the food moves through your stomach and intestines? All of these depend on what is consumed with what.

4. Forget about losing weight with a diet. Think about eating for optimal health, energy and improved quality of life. You will naturally lose weight to the appropriate level based on your body and its needs.

5. Remember being skinny is not a sign of being healthy. Skinny people also have diseases and health complaints related to how they eat. You should aim to be healthy while being of good weight while giving your body nutrient-dense food.

ALSO: -

1. **Carbs:-** These feed your brain. Avoiding them will diminish your brain power. You can choose to eat complex carbohydrates. (whole grains, fruit and veggies) Simple carbs are not healthy period. They breakdown too quickly and cause spikes in blood

sugar which causes weight gain. Plus, you will continue indulging in these with constant cravings.

2. **Fats**:- Fats do not cause you to gain weight unless you over eat in an abundance.

3. **Blood Sugar and Glycemic Load**: - This is how quickly or slowly the breaks down food, converts it to sugar or either uses it or stores it into fat. The more a food is processed or has sugar added the worse it is. Ideally, you want to break down food slowly and use as fuel as you go. Weight gain happens when the body stores unused food as fat or when too much insulin is released. Do not make poor food choices.

4. **Fat Burning Foods, Good For Weight Loss**:-
This all depends on a properly working metabolism. That is the process of converting food to fuel. Some people are naturally lean, they have a "fast metabolism". Others seem to smell a donut and gain weight. They have a "slow metabolism". You need to maintain your metabolism by finding out the things that slow down your metabolism.

7. **Five Ways You Can Recognize**: -

1. **Low Levels of Activity:** Healthy weight depends on how much you move to increase heat to burn calories and invigorate digestion to breakdown food.

2.**The Gradual Loss of Lean Tissue, From Lack of Exercise**: Muscle weighs more than fat. Muscle also helps burn fat. You have to increase muscle tone. This can be done by walking, using light hand weights. Doing simple chores like vacuuming, alternate hands. Also, activities like mowing the lawn.

3. Not Eating Regular, Well-Balanced Meals:-
Every time you eat your metabolism is jump started. Food is fuel and eating starts the process for body to breakdown, digest and eliminate. Not eating sends the body into starvation mode where it begins storing fat.

4. Fasting Or Dieting That Restricts Caloric Intake, For Extended Periods:- This is so bad for you. It deprives the body of essential nutrients that are needed for survival. Restricting calories depletes lean muscle tissue. When diet is over people tend to overeat to compensate.

5. Insufficient Daily Protein, Consumption:-
Consume protein every day whether animal of plant variety. It provides body with energy and burns slower than carbohydrates, this extends energy and stabilizes blood sugar levels.

Balancing these five issues will help you balance your metabolism. A faster metabolism will help you reach and maintain an ideal weight and ratio of fat to muscle.

8. **There are six ways to Improve Your Metabolism: Weight and Strength Training**:- This will increase muscle tissue. The more muscle you have, the more calories you will burn throughout the day.

1. **Regular Physical Activity**:- This will turn up the heat and melt fat and calories away. Regular fitness is best but even walking, raking leaves, or even housework at a faster pace can burn calories.

2. **Keep Hormones And Blood Sugar Levels Stable**:- Consume whole grains and low sugar foods while decreasing toxic preservative intake. Take supplements.

3. **Drink Plenty of Water**:- This keep the system working. Water can flush toxins that make the metabolism sluggish.

4. **Eat Smaller Meals And Snack More Often**:- Consume a snack like a piece of fruit or nuts every 3 hours. This will help maintain a steady level of energy and keep blood sugar levels from dropping. When it does drop, unhealthy food cravings emerge.

5. **Eat Foods That Stoke Your Metabolism**:-Yes, there are foods that actually play into your metabolism. They stoke up your internal temperature. Improve breakdown of food and fat, plus remove toxins and increase metabolism.

This list includes Drinks/Foods/Spices/Supplements.

1. Drinks:- Drink a bottle of ice water every day. Do not drink with food. Also drink that Green Tea. This will eliminate toxins and increase metabolism.

2. **Foods:-** Eat plenty of protein for energy. And whole grain carbs. This helps to maintain energy, blood sugar levels and elimination schedules. The grins remove cholesterol from the blood and help maintain bowel function. The protein gives you sustained energy for exercise.

3. **Spices**:-Include chilli, mustard, allspice, ginger, garlic, onion, curries, turmeric, cloves, cayenne. Pick what you like. This can speed up your metabolism roughly 40% for the next two hours after ingesting.

1. Food is a critical piece of the wellness puzzle.

2.Food can cause pain, inflammation and affect joints due to having excess weight.

3. A typical American diet is filled with saturated fats and trans fats, sugars, preservatives, convenience food, and overly processed food. This is a deadly recipe for acidity, inflammation and pain.
4. Avoid inflammatory foods and consume as much fresh, organic, whole foods as possible.

5. Eating a diet rich in anti-inflammatory foods, filled with dense nutrients, can reduce pain, inflammation and body mass.
6. Essential to keep green tea, mushrooms, turmeric and water in your diet. They all reduce inflammation and pain,
7. Forget diets, forget counting carbs and calories. Stick to basic healthy eating. Stabilize your blood sugar by learning about the glycemic load of everything you eat and consume metabolism boosting foods and spices. You will be the weight you are meant to be!

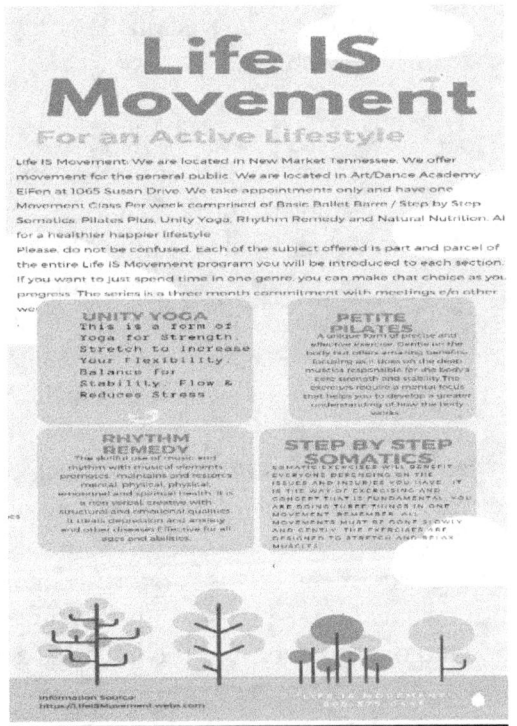

WRAP- UP

This book and others are written with the hopes that dancers will get more educated and not just look at the instant fluff of belly dancing. Now we turn our attention to not the needs of dancers but every human being. Sharing this knowledge has taken years of training as a dancer and investigating why things go wrong. I have learned a great deal from all the students who have passed through my studio doors from New England to Southern CA and here in Eastern Tennessee. They have sparked my interest.

As I have grown older and over worked my own body, I realized I needed help. On moving from California my husband was diagnosed as diabetic. Several things in our life changed. I have arthritis, peripheral neuropathy. We have always eaten well and felt it was a healthy diet. We have made changes and delved back into practice and things studied and put in the past. So, the last 4 years or so have brought us to the point where we are today. The information that we have, is being shared. We have expanded our practice to include the general public who can benefit from movement and added these other benefits too. Our new area, as you can imagine is called "Life IS Movement".

We both have been blessed to have wonderful careers and hope and pray to be able to continue sharing what we know with others. Dance and Music is where it is at! We are not just training dancers and musicians but also sharing our methods to the general public to benefit their health, whatever it may be.

Thank you,   Morwenna Assaf

Walid Assaf

https://DancerAndDrummer.webs.com

https://LifeISMovement.webs.com

Other books authored by
Morwenna Assaf

1. *Finger Cymbals: Play Them Correctly

2. *ZILLS-ZAGAT Teachers Syllabus

3. *Handbook of Dance Terminology*
Dictionary of Vocabulary for Middle Eastern Dance Studies

3. *The Experience of Theater Dance For "Belly Dancers"
4. ** Mosaic of Music: The Mystery of Percussion and Dance"
5. Creativity: THE POWER OF COMMITMENT
Creativity – Get Going
Creativity – Find Your Stride
Creativity – Establish Visibility
Creativity – Success! The Finish Line

6. *Shiny Beads and Shimmies*
Welcome to Belly Dance/Ask Before You Undulate

7. *Academic approach to Arabic Dance*
For Belly Dancers Who Want To Teach

8. *The Art of Teaching Oriental Danse*
Teach With Authority and Know-How!
9. *Performing Your Best As A Middle
Eastern Dance Artist*
Be The Best You Can!

Upcoming Books to Be Published by
August 2018
1. Threads of Identity
2. Ancient Whisperings
3. BOBBY Says

CDs & DVDs offered through
CEDAR Productions

CD = Art/Dance Academy Warm-Up
Music
Art/Dance Academy Basic Rhythms
Art/Dance Academy Advanced
Rhythms
Soiree Orientale
Ancient Whisperings - Music of
Phoenicia
Eastern Bedouin Favorites

DVD = Practice for Belly Dancers

Classes and Coaching are held at
Art/Dance Academy

FOR ALL Levels and Non-Dancers

Contact Art/Dance Academy @ 865-
375-0446

ArabiDanseAcademeie@sbcglobal.net

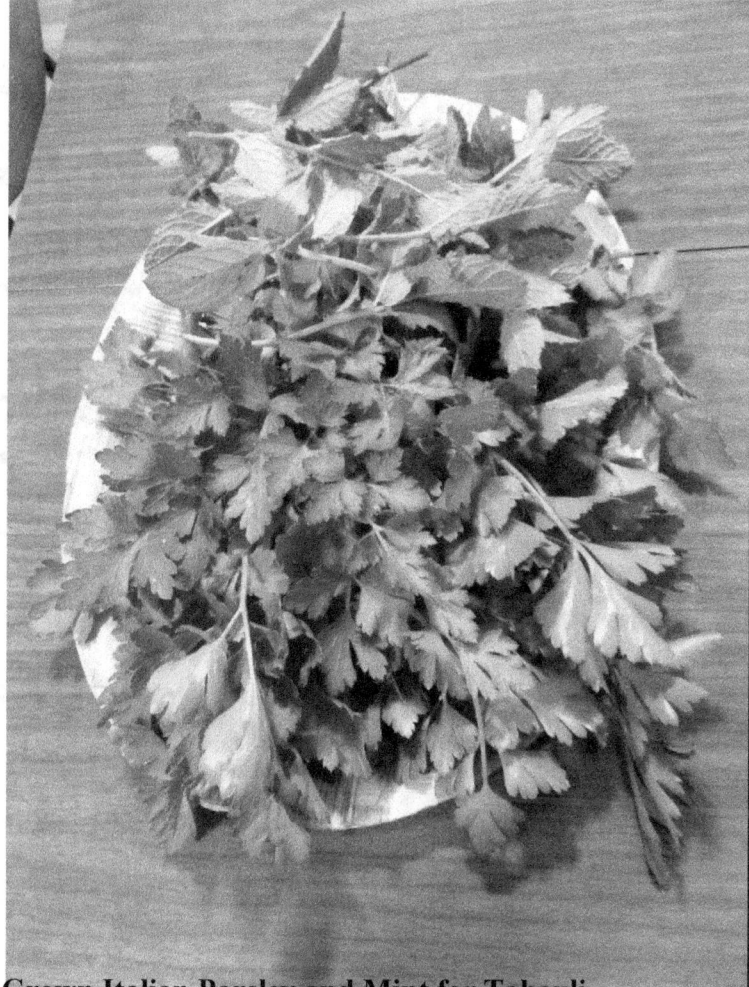

Home Grown Italian Parsley and Mint for Tabouli.

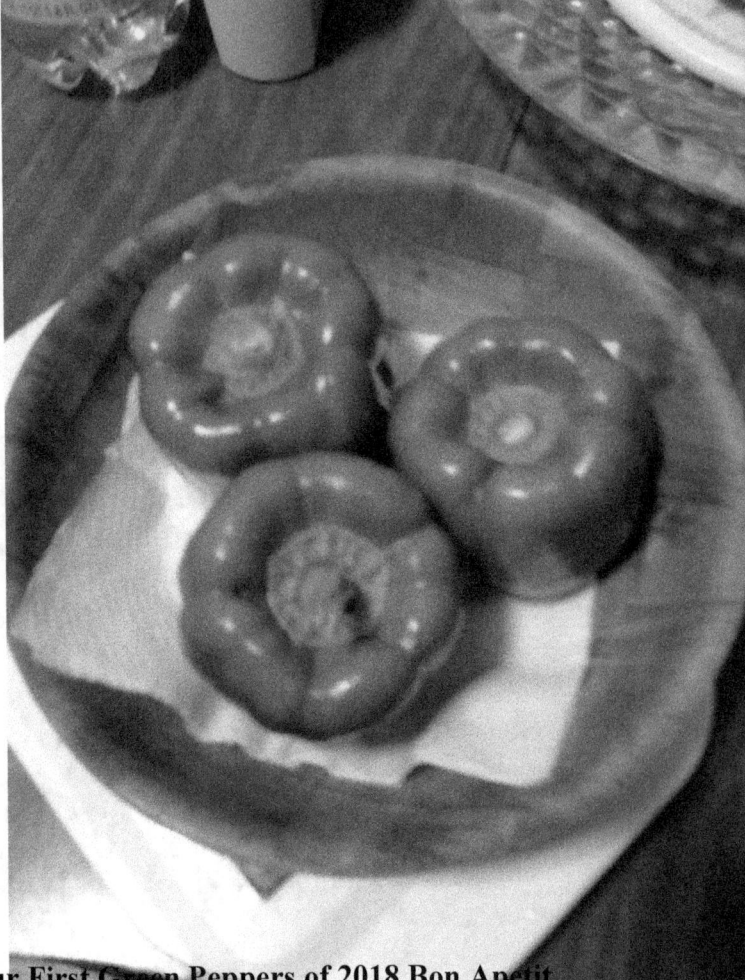

Our First Green Peppers of 2018 Bon Apetit

www.ingramcontent.com/pod-product-compliance
Lightning Source LLC
Chambersburg PA
CBHW071209280526
45787CB00002B/622